A NOT
SO FINE
MADNESS

Adele T. Stewart

A NOT SO FINE MADNESS

ISBN-978-1-4092-2465-5

For my husband,
who gave me a chance.
Not once,
. . . Endlessly.

&

For my mother,
who validates love,
. . . Completely.

FOREWORD

Have you ever seen a major car park in your city, with the huge neon sign above it flashing "FULL"?

Well, then you may begin to understand what the brain of a person that deals with manic depression (bipolar) may be experiencing.

If you replace "cars" with "messages" it's like this....

Our minds are over-crowded with double-parked thoughts. There are queues of incoming and outgoing messages waiting to be processed, with the variety of feelings to go with it...aggravation, impatience, untroubled, happy, exhaustion, ecstatic, and more...messages that weave in and out and around other messages, others that are jammed in reverse, and others that can't find the brake pedal too!

What chaos!

Hope you are able to see through the window of my life. It may help you deal with your mum, dad, sibling, child, friend. Or just find comfort knowing maybe why your loved one died from this debilitating illness, or just for you, yourself a fellow sufferer.

The writing style I have used is not that of traditional ways. It does not have flow, so if you feel you cant see the story flow, it won't. I go back and forth with story. So each chapter is basically like a point. It has a heading to go with that thought, and it can also have things that I have already brought up before, but this is because it relates to the chapter heading and incidents again.

So, come in, sit down, hold tight and join me on my life's roller coaster...

"I doubt sometimes whether a quiet
and unagitated life would have suited me
- yet I sometimes long for it."

- Byron

CONTENTS

1. The First Meltdown

2. The Missing Piece of the Puzzle.

3. Culminated Result

4. A Brief Memory Of Early Childhood

5. Homemade Family

6. Post-natal Depression?

7. May May Mania!!!

8. My Instincts Proved Me Right

9. Moved By Reading

10. The Dangerous Stoops In The Highs

11. Betrayal and Depression

12. That Fear of Lost Friends Rears its Ugly Head

13. The $650 Ride

14. Comfort in Other Sufferers' Stories

15. Dr. Rejection

16. It's Enough to Make You Pull your Hair Out

17. Trichotillomania

18. Life Coach

19. Meds, Meds, Meds!

20. It's No Wonder I'm Crazy!!!!

21. Feel Like Fishing

22. Dedication, Nurture and Love

23.   Looking Through the Window of Rage

24.   What is Tolerable or Acceptable?

25.   Coming to Terms

26.   Clinical Terminologies

27.   Clarifying the Label

28.   Restructuring Thoughts and Behaviours

29.   Tock-Tick!

30.   Hereditary Genealogy

31.   Where in the Brain Does Bipolar Form?

32.   Through My Children's Eyes

33.   To Those on The Other Side

34.   Who Am I, Who Should I Be?

35.   Looking for Light at the End of the Tunnel

36.   Sunny Bear Polar Bear

37.   The Fine Balance

38.   Survival at its Best

39.   Advice for My Friends When I Awaken & Fall Into The Darkness!

40.   Needing To Be Needed

41.   Die –Eat

42.   The No-No's

43.   A Cherished Experience

44.   The Past, The Present, The Future

1. THE FIRST MELTDOWN

For many people, I know their first job is the best time of their lives; becoming independent, having a wage, not having time schedules for assignments to be handed in, no more homework and being able to have your own money to decide to spend it how you wish! Basically this is called *independence*. Although this is partly inconceivable to me, my first job was for the most part, a terrible struggle. I was almost fourteen years old and didn't really want to leave school so young. I was starting to really enjoy my curriculum. But my parents saw fit for me to start work then. I actually had my heart set on being a dental nurse at the end of that year.

Sometimes I had months of great fun, passion, high enthusiasm, and long runs of very hard but enjoyable work. And then I lost all interest in my work, friends, and life. I had no idea what was happening to me and I would wake up in the morning with a profound sense of dread that I was going to have to somehow make it through another entire day. To take a break, I would go the toilet, but was then unable to muster enough energy to go back typing. I would stare out the glass front doors, stare at my computer screen, shuffle, rearrange my typing jobs for the day until the girl training me would get cross and continually tell me to get on with it. I have very few good memories from this job, some rather, shall I say unfortunate things occurred to me, for someone that was a young, naïve and pretty girl back then. Unfortunately, I was employed by a man, who used his power and stance to take advantage of the young and innocent. He thought he would get away with inappropriate behaviour such as touching girls in the wrong places, and not use appropriate conversation in the work environment. He expected to be treated in a special way, and had requests that made me feel awkward and against my will. Every morning, we were to greet him (boss) with a kiss!! (Yeah! WHAT?!.. not a criteria I would expect as the norm looking back now). He was triple my age, and I felt very special that my boss would have me at his best interests, but when I got fed up with it, it seemed that I was exaggerating and trying to cause problems! He is known as a meddler, and gets away with his actions to this very day. I am glad he has no part of my life in any way.

During and around this time frame, someone close to our family had been diagnosed with *papilloma virus (* see below). It was awful! I enquired how this would have occurred. As the symptoms and explanations were being verbalised, I fell into what seemed like a deep trance... my eyes were open, but all I saw was black. Spiralling thoughts whooshed around my brain, I became limp in my limbs, and couldn't stay standing up. As memories came flooding in, I felt sick and panic run through my veins. I shook uncontrollably. I was awake and reliving a awful childhood memory, that wasn't part of my existence until this very moment. It must have been buried deep in my subconscious right until now. Remembering the time I was wheeled down a dark corridor, my little body on this big metal bed of white stiff cold sheets…I would ask, "Mummy, what's happening?".

Now it made sense. I too was also exposed to this virus. I was only five or six at the time.

Even more memories came flooding into my mind, memories of sexual interference, and one occasion in particular. Yes, now things were adding up to be clearer, I was putting 2 and 2 together…I couldn't believe that I had never remembered this before now! The operations, the awkward embarrassment of people I never knew touching me in places that I had been taught were private.

Before I knew it, a mask was over my little nose and mouth, and I fell asleep. When I awoke, my private parts were burning; I sobbed and asked "What happened Mummy?" She just held my little hand, and said something to the effect, that the Dr. had to fix something to make me better. I actually don't even know if she herself knew how I contracted the virus.

The memories, horrid memories, were all too much to bear. I went into a meltdown. I was shaking, barely keeping down the substances that were in my stomach. I cried and cried inconsolably! I started hyperventilating into the first one of my many panic attack episodes that was to follow! I cannot remember the circumstances as to why and where I was when all this was internally revealed

I was mad! How was I going to deal with this!? At this stage of my life, I was a teenager following a path as a Christian. Was I to bury it and move on! I couldn't bear talking to my parents about it! It would destroy all of us!

* *Genital warts-- These are growths that appear around the genitals or anus, and sometimes in the vagina, rectum or urethra.*

Transmission-- About one-third of the HPV types can be spread through sexual contact. Warts may take a few weeks to many months (or even years) to appear.

Treatment--Warts are frozen by applying liquid nitrogen or dry ice once a week. It usually takes several applications before the warts disappear. Also Laser treatment is used when warts are in places that are difficult to reach, very extensive or resistant to other treatments. Laser treatment is administered in hospital under a general anaesthetic.

Recurrence-- After treatment-most treatments destroy cells that are infected by the wart virus. In most people, warts go away eventually and do not reappear. This is thought to be due to the body's natural defences. Genital warts can be managed. With patience and persistence, the warts will go away.

2. THE MISSING PIECE OF THE PUZZLE

So, you are probably on the end of your seat…. What happened - you say. Those memories I was having was of when I was around 5, but no more than 7.

I don't recall it as rape. It didn't involve intercourse, and it definitely wasn't under threatening circumstances. With a more advance knowledge of the situation now, I know it as "groomed". So what is grooming? Is it not as serious as other types of abuse? I decided to do my own research and came up with the following results…

HOW GROOMING TRANSPIRES

Lloyd Sinclair, MSSW
Midwest Centre for Psychotherapy and Sex Therapy
[Biographical notes]

- Behaviour to Gain Trust
- Reassuring to the Family
- Gradual Erosion of Boundaries
- Construct Secrecy With Child
- Working to Secure Compliance

Mr. Sinclair comments: "In the context of the sexual molestation of children, the term grooming may seem incongruous. Yet the closest familiar analogue to grooming is the common ritual of courting.
How do child molesters groom potential victims? Like the man engaged in courting, the child molester behaves in ways to promote trust; and since the victim is often a part of a family, he will also try to gain the trust of the child's parents or care-providers. Child molesters often select their potential victims carefully, typically targeting the child who is seeking adult attention. Most often there is some period before the molester engages in any inappropriate behaviour. During this time, the molester presents himself positively to the child, exhibits interest, is complimentary, and behaves in exemplary ways to reassure anyone who may be suspicious of his motives.
Once trust is accomplished, the child molester will begin to test and erode typical boundaries to sexual behaviour. He might suggest that the child and he sleep in the same bed, be nude together, or he may touch the child near the genital area to test the child's reaction. He may suggest that the child engage in non-sexual inappropriate behaviour such as drinking alcohol, in order to make the child fearful that he or she will be in trouble if their activities together are discovered.
If the child does not appear overly upset or report these boundary violations to others, then the molester might escalate the intrusiveness of his sexual behaviours. Ultimately, the goal of grooming is to obtain compliance so the child will be available for sexual abuse.
For example, the child molester frequently will tell the child that touching between them is good, that it is an indication of their special relationship, and that if the child reports the behaviour they will no longer be able to be friends. Some molesters threaten, and tell the child that by not complying with the touching the child, or some person important to the child, will be harmed.

If a man is interested in having sex with a woman, he knows success is unlikely if he simply approaches her and suggests sex. Instead, he will present his positive attributes and himself as someone interested in her. Often he will seek to gain the trust and approval of her friends and family. Frequently the courtship process is reciprocal, each actively courting the other.

Similarly, grooming behaviours employed by sex offenders are intended to increase the likelihood of success in engaging a child in sexual behaviour. Of course, preventing the child from telling someone is one goal not generally related to adult courtship.

The fundamental distinction, however, between child molestation and courtship is that children cannot consent to sexual activity with adults. The legal bar to a child's consent is recognition of the lack of information and power a child has in a sexual relationship with an adult. Therefore, there can be no reciprocity.

In courting behaviour, the intended target of the sexual behaviour has equality of knowledge and power with the person who is seeking to have sex. Grooming a child, on the other hand, is manipulation of an uninformed relatively powerless victim. Children are especially at risk due to their lack of understanding about the motives behind the acts of adults directed toward sex. Children's lack of understanding renders them extremely vulnerable to adult advances."

So here you have it. I was basically a baby, and a man of whom our family trusted took advantage of my innocence. It was clear to me now, after many thoughts and recollections, that he may not have purposely done these things. I don't believe it was pre-meditated. Actually, I think that intoxication could have played a big part in his actions. But putting this aside, it is not an excuse for him at all! And now that I have the memories of the incidents, I see a grown irresponsible individual of whom was for putting himself in this situation! It was now something else to deal with, and most likely the reason for many things that have occurred to me in my life. Thus, the missing piece of the puzzle. I have had a very big problem with instability and fear of losing loved ones all of my life, and have also had problems with self esteem. I have never learnt to treat myself right. I place all my attention on all the other people I cherish in my life and forget about me. But "what about me", I say; I'm just a human, vulnerable to other people's fantasies and lack of control! I have felt used and abused, and therefore have grown to think of myself in this way. If I was popular and liked for this, I would allow it. It was a form of stability for me.

As my writing progresses, you will see that I have been working on mending my inner thoughts and self esteem, but so much has had to transpire before I have come to that!

3. CULMINATED RESULT

From this time on, I had this pattern of shifting moods and energies which had a very seductive side. To a large extent, I experienced intoxicatingly high moods that would help me to forget the terror that lay inside me. I wanted the floating feeling to stay; everything was all right when these came about. These generated more than enough energy to give me at least the illusion of managing everything in excess. Buying just one small gift of appreciation for a colleague would result in buying two or three. Instead of buying a single cassette of the song that I loved and had heard on the radio, I would buy the whole album of the singer, and a couple other cassettes while I was at it, even knowing I had other things intended to be paid for with my wages that week. I would buy things "in case" I ran out of items, or "if I need them down the track" type of attitude. I had and have a magnetic attraction to specials and sales. The thought that I could save money on a full priced item, but really, in the end, spend more than I would if I had just perhaps bought the one dinner set or the one set of glasses for my glory box. I would get three or four sets in case in 10 years time the pattern would be outdated perhaps, and my settings would be incomplete!!

My passion is craft. I would also spend hours and hours making things for people - brooches out of Fimo (a cookable colourful clay), photo frames, gift packages, and I would even sew little skirts and bibs for the young ones in our church community. I loved giving people these gifts. In moments of deep soul searching I would craft emotional words, poems or letters about any little thing I thought was important or special to me at the time, and I would outpour the sentiments onto paper. This gave me a sense of stability. I thought I was safe if I could be surrounded by people who appreciated me and my kindness, and I had a wall to lean on when I fell apart. Sometimes the gifts were a way of saying *sorry* for what I might have done to upset them through my irritability or highly energetic spurts. I felt insecure that I was going to lose friends and have no one around.

I was a single child till I was eleven, happy, smiley and polite. Deep inside though, was another matter from what was showing on the outside. I didn't know at all what these moods were. To me, it was just part of puberty and adolescence, with added stressors of an unsettled family lifestyle.

4. A BRIEF MEMORY OF EARLY CHILDHOOD

I loved my father. He was one of two major people in my life as a single child. He called me his "chicken little". Because I was the only child at this time at home, I was given a lot of attention. The time that dad put into my young days have made a big influence on me to my adult days. Dad was a very hands-on man. He managed a beautiful garden, and taught me how to plant, weed, and look after many different areas of it. I remember him making a special plot just for me to take care of. He gently encouraged me how to keep up the care of it. He was a very busy dad as I remember. He ran his own huge business, and had many employees of a large painting firm. Many times, when he came home at night, and he had to prepare to the next days job, I would sit in the shed on a paint pot chatting to him. He would explain to me what he was doing, and give me little errands to help him. I never felt threatened by him during these times. We had a closeness, and I felt loved and protected by him. He had a soft spot for animals, particularly dogs (which is where I'm sure I too have adopted the same admiration for them). I always had a pet in my home life.

On the other hand, dad had another side which was dark, irritable and intolerant. He had a intolerance of noise, nonsense and uncleanliness (particularly dusty surfaces). This other side revealed a very bad temper. He was verbally and physically abusive during this so called "bad time". He was scary. These spurts were unpredictable, and shocking. It became a normal part of my life.

Thankfully, my mother was my shelter. She was there to hold me. Quite often the scenario was of Dad screaming outside a locked bedroom door. I would cry in fear of the unknown, and I know mum too was holding back her tears, but her bravery was for my fear.

During my early school years, there would be times mum would pick me up in the middle of the day, and we would go for a drive. Usually it would be to my grandparents' home. She had our things packed, and we would stay for a couple of days. My mum was accustomed to wearing sunglasses even if it wasn't a sunny day. Now I know it was to hide the fact that she had been crying. Dad had also hit her in his rages. She protected me as much as she could by keeping me away from the home while dad was like this.

One of my fondest memories was when she would take me shopping. As a child, I would forget what had happened for a while. We would share a cappuccino and pieces of spice toast cut into triangles, smothered in butter every time (I can still smell it, as I recall it).

She would take me to the park and let me play for hours, swing me on the swings, play chasey and chat. (From old home movies I have seen, I gather I was a hyperactive child and couldn't sit still for long periods; therefore the park would have obviously been a good alternative while she tried to calm her nerves from dad's tempers). In the park I could run free, unlike at home where I could wreak havoc or provoke dad any further!

Mum was sweet, affectionate and calm in front of me as much as possible. We did lots together. Another very fond memory I have was when mum and I were watching TV together. I would get my doll clothes and dress her feet and we would pretend to have conversations between the four of us, and make up funny scenarios (this is most likely where my twisted humour and imagination have stemmed from!!!).

But there were times dad would threaten to take me away from her, and I would tense up inside my little body in fear that I would never see her again! At those times she would argue and fight for me. I was between two parents I dearly loved and knew no other way than to love the two equally. Therefore the thought of whom I would rather be with, was inconceivable and impossible.. Yet my emotions were forced into choosing between the two. All I wanted was for all three of us to be together and for us to all be happy.

In the quiet, peaceful, happy home life stages, dad took on the duty to sit by my bedside reading *Blinky Bill* while I was dozing off to sleep. During occasional meal times my dad would do funny tricks with his two dessert spoons and sing songs along to the clicking of the beat he made with them! He loved to tease me with hiding a coin behind my ear, and taking it from my other ear! They laughed with my frustration, as I couldn't figure it out! He taught me how to eat with chopsticks before I was five, with my breakfast cereal! His passion was fishing. And on the long trips he was away, I loved waiting for him to come home, knowing he would explain all the different types of things he caught. I watched his skills in cleaning them with mum, and basically with everything dad did, he would always explain and educate you in the basics of life! (the bad part of the fishing trips resulted in the scraps being made into a YUCKY fish soup I was forced to try, while I was gagging! Yuccck!). On the other hand, they would spoil me to the extreme. I had the most memorable birthday parties. Lots of my friends came. Mum and dad would dress me up all pretty, I would have a huge cake, lots of colourful balloons and streamers and everything those days was just the greatest. Lots of toys, a beautiful bedroom, and I was always dressed lovely. Christmas times were my favourite times of the year, and like any other home life, I helped set up the tree, and the nativity setting. On Christmas Eve, dad was responsible in helping me leave the carrot and milk out for Santa. Dad and mum were accustomed to "doing it big!". All their friends, family and employees were invited for the Christmas Party. I would dance and play with my cousins and children of their friends. I would get a new special dress too for these times. One particular Christmas, I got my very first bike. My dad spent many hours patiently teaching me to pedal and steer! It had a white basket on the front with a flower! I just loved it. Finally I learnt to ride without my trainer wheels, and when dad was outside I was allowed to ride up and down the street paths, showing how clever I was!

As for my view of my parents' relationship as a child, I would be happy when dad would spoil my mum with flowers and gifts. I think these were times a child would consider that they had made up, and I was happy because of this. It would help me feel secure between the storms.

So, these are just some of my memories up to the age of eight. And for me, in a child's view of things, they were mostly happy, healthy times.

5. HOMEMADE FAMILY

As the years went by, I reached the age when serious dating was permissible.

There was at our church an attraction I had to a quiet, tall dark and handsome guy. He drove a LOUD, bright blue 'XY Falcon'.

I finally got the courage to talk to him, and with the help of some very dear friends of ours, we were able to spend more time with each other by going to their home for suppers. Eventually, I realised he was all I needed in my life. He listened and cared for me when things at home were upsetting. I confided in him all my fears, and told him all about my history. I felt secure in his arms. He was my protection! He was the one to rescue me. God did bless me, and we were married. I was nineteen, and rather young. He was three years older. I wanted children straightaway. But he wasn't too keen with the idea. But eight months after we were married I fell pregnant. At the time, I was working as switchboard operator for a new car sales company. It was stressful, the boss was awful, and I was very tired. At the end of the day I was irritable. Seven weeks into the pregnancy I lost the baby. I understood very little of what was going on and felt that only death would release me from the overwhelming sense of inadequacy and blackness that surrounded me. I felt utterly alone and thought I'd never ever be able to carry any more babies. I had a curette, and the doctor told us to wait for three months before trying again. We did and I fell pregnant immediately. The pregnancy was good, although I was very vulnerable, sensitive and teary. We were blessed with a very healthy baby boy, bright, playful and smiley!

My first weeks as a mother were just overwhelming, and as any parent would know, you watch every movement they make, you smell their skin, you kiss their little velvet lips and feel so blessed that you could both produce such an awesome being!

He was a hard baby to breastfeed. He lost weight and after four weeks the paediatrician resorted to placing him on the bottle. He also didn't sleep much. Although that didn't seem to trouble him, we did the normal tests for lactose intolerance, etc. He was pale and continued losing weight. We found that he was anaemic. We were advised to add vitamins to his formula. We would take it in turns feeding him during the night.

At this stage, I was fatigued through lack of sleep. He would only sleep an hour at a time, and would be aroused by the slightest noise! He was a wriggly bubs while asleep and we consistently hung our hands over the bed to rock the bassinette, in case he awoke!

6. POST-NATAL DEPRESSION?

When our son was six months old, we travelled to Melbourne for a holiday. It was fun showing off our new baby to family and friends over there. On the other hand, I experienced a rather erratic mood change! It was more severe in comparison with my teenage years, and we put it down to just having had a baby, and lack of sleep. Both could have been true, but looking back now, it was the beginning of what I now know to be *manic depression*!

This little baby boy continued to be so active that he wouldn't keep still. Before he could even crawl, when he sat on the floor, he had the habit of laughing and throwing himself back with such force that he'd almost knock himself out on the surface behind him. So we always constructed a barricade of pillows around him. But he did the same when he was being held, and would head-butt us with such force that he made us see stars!

One particular night in Melbourne was the **beginning** of what I call **'the rest of my life revelation'**…

Our baby would not sleep and I was making tea. It was rather late. I was tired and hungry and the baby didn't eat his solids for me. What he did eat ended up all over my shoulder! I was irritable and argued with my husband - what we argued about, I wouldn't have a clue! All I remember is that I was at one side of the bedroom and my husband was on the other. I **threw** the baby at him and said I was leaving and never coming back. I'd had enough, and couldn't handle all the pressure any more.

I grabbed the car keys, burnt the wheels out down the drive and sped off with such a careless speed. I drove and drove and drove… I didn't know where I was going; it was night time, lights just flashed past me in blurs, and I didn't know where anything was. This was the first time I had ever been to Melbourne in my life! I went through red stop lights and swerved all over the road, howling my head off and hoping to hit something so I would be killed. I felt helpless and hopeless. Ahead was a sign '24 HOUR MEDICAL CENTRE'. I swerved into the entrance, parked the car and staggered into Reception, asking to see a doctor as soon as possible. All that was going through my head was, *"I'm acting like my father. I've gone completely mad! I must be schizophrenic or have manic depression!"* (When I lived at home, Mum and I always wondered whether dad had one of these illnesses after we had read articles about them.) That night, the words I read in these articles went over and over in my mind. And I finally figured I must have Dad's genes and was completely insane!

As the doctor called me into his office, I remember not feeling at all comfortable with him. He seemed unconcerned about my demeanour, and as I blubbered my way through expressing fears of having manic depression like my dad, he assured me it wasn't hereditary. He said I was only acting this way because I had grown up watching the way dad was, and was only mimicking his actions. I believed this to be true fact!

The years from 8-19 were very difficult for me. Sometimes life at home was unbearable. I was a tense, stressed and on edge teenager. My appetite was that of a bird (as my husbands mother use to say). Because as I have already described in chapter 4, my fathers shifting mood swings never got any better. It was a fearful scenario a lot of the time. To just go to school or work was a relief, to have the 6-8 hours in a normal environment. But concerns were always left with my mums' safety, and she would be in the back of my mind. Getting engaged and married was what I wanted for a while. It was like a chain was cut. I felt guilt on the other hand though, leaving my mum and sister. I seemed to have grown into the child that had to intervene between the shocking times. I had to yell to get dads attention to separate rages and physical manias of his. It had formed me into being a nervous wreck. My emotions were toyed with. I seemed to live with two lives. The one, a happy content and unagitated Christian lifestyle, and then on the other hand, the abusive, screaming, fearful life of a manic depressive father.

We tried to gently approach him in his quiet moods and reason with him that he needed help, but that never eventuated due to denial of the problem.

So, here I was, I felt totally humiliated and all I thought of was how weak and jelly-spined I was, **copying my dad's habits**, the habits I hated so much! What had come over me? I left the surgery and was glad I was to never visit that doctor again. I took a deep breath, and vowed to pull myself together. I would recheck every thing I did, making sure I wasn't like my dad, but I couldn't help it!

As I drove back to the place where we were staying, I fell into a deep, mesmerised state. I was exhausted and confused about myself. I expressed remorse for my actions to my husband, and crawled into bed to hopefully sleep the night's dramas away, hoping for a fresh new start in the morning.

7. "MAY"NIA !!!

I had developed a bad temper and was very emotional! I had crazy highs.

When I was eight months pregnant with our second baby, I recall planting lawn in the back and front of our home. It was already grown lawn, which you cut into squares and plugged into the soil, evenly spaced so it would then spread and grow together. The area I did was well over 144 square metres combining front and back yards. Basically, I would suggest there was nothing wrong with this under normal circumstances, other than the fact I started at sunrise and went till I had finished, needing the help of the porch lights to complete it! The intense, continual bending over caused my breeched eight-month baby to do a complete turn and face head down!!!! (I wouldn't recommend this procedure to those carrying breech!!)

I also continued to have massive high energy shopping sprees where I'd spend all the grocery money that was budgeted for the nappies and formula. Instead, I'd spend it on silly things that I thought were very important at the time, because they were on special, and that I would be able to store them away for times we would need them. I'd buy shoes or clothing that had been on Sale racks! At these fantastic times, I'd be ultra-friendly to anyone at the shops. I'd stop to chat and ask strangers all about themselves, or their children, then go on my way! I would have the housework totally up to date, dinner made. Somehow, the month of **May** always seemed to be my happy period. Maybe it was the calm before the storms of deep black winters, although I couldn't really call it "the calm", seeing my happy times were ecstatically happy. Sometimes I would just bake for days. I would freeze meals, cakes, biscuits etc for when we would have visitors over and sometimes take meals to others that were struggling, and help out with their house work as well!

I would sit for hours painting window glass art with the boys when they were kindy age. I would stock up on making supplies of scrap booking cards, paint jars, tee-shirts, pillow covers etc etc. BUT, these fun times were also shared with periods of total despair, made even worse by terrible agitation. My mind would race from subject to subject, and instead of being filled with the excited and powerful thoughts associated with earlier periods of rapid thinking, I became exceedingly restless, angry and irritable. The only way I could tame the agitation was to keep busy. I would lay in my bed trying to sleep, and then have a fantastic idea to clean a room in the house or I would plan what venture I was going on the next morning. Once I dug a huge fish pond in our back yard, all done and completed by that night, with water, fish and fountain (the fish never survived though, I never let them adjust to the water like you are meant too!!!). My husband would come home to find that I had abandoned all the normal duties of the house since he'd left that morning for work. His left over remains of cut lunch and breakfast were still on the sink, beds unmade, children still in PJs, and bank depleted of funds once again. I had no idea what was going on and felt totally unable to ask anyone for help. It never occurred to me that I was ill! After all, the Melbourne doctor had reassured me I wasn't!!!!!

By the weekends, I was usually exhausted. My husband would then have to take over as I slept the days away. When I was sitting in our seats at church, I would go into a mesmerised stare and it was like watching the animated conversations between members. It was a blur, and I would only respond to greetings with the same typical façade, daring to not show the crazy emotions externally of what I was feeling internally! I was just too exhausted to respond. These times gradually moved into the next state…depression. I stopped answering the phone and took hot baths in the vain hope that I might somehow escape from the deadness and dreariness. I'd be drenched by awful sounds and images! I'd see myself jumping in front of semi-trailers and dying! Or I'd imagine emptying my medicine cupboard and consuming copious amounts of medication with a glass of port to slow down my brain and stop the cogs spinning for a while just to let me sleep.

But as the depression deepened, all I did was sleep. My body ached all over, my joints were sore. I barely managed to get up to go to the toilet. The door of my room was kept closed and I was slipping into a different world. What happened outside the door didn't concern me in the least.

8. MY INSTINCTS PROVED ME RIGHT

Things went on like this for another few years. Eventually the depression went away of its own accord. But in due course, it would regroup and mobilize for the next attack. Just as night certainly follows day, my mood would crash, and my mind again would grind to a halt. Violent and dreadful nightmares recurred. My moods shifted week by week. .

I remember when we were in need of money, that I would put my craftiness into work! I hired a market stall weekly, and sold hand-painted T-shirts and windcheaters.

I would stay up night after night, hour after hour, hand painting children's size T-shirts with copied cartoon characters from colouring in books, and then sold them and took orders every Thursday and Friday. I would put my two little boys into child care twice a week so I could accomplish this, just for enough money to cover groceries and petrol for the week. At the same time my husband would come home from his full time job, and go and deliver pizzas for extra money as well. Yes, we were in a pickle! This went on for weeks. Sometimes he wouldn't be awake enough to go and deliver, so I would take the toddlers, and deliver for him for an hour or two so he could have a sleep first before the long night ahead of him. I remember feeding my two littlies garlic bread, to keep them content whilst I drove around.

Another time, a few years on, I decided I was going to do the yellow pages round. ALL ON MY OWN! This was in a splurge of a MASSIVE high. And I imagined I would cope fine doing this for the seven days to complete it in. Two of our three children were then at school. I remember going to my parents' house to pick up the trailer, and then going to the depot to pick up the huge pallet of over a thousand fat, yellow, shrink wrapped books. I borrowed a trolley, and off I went. The area I was given was a partly industrial area, with major roads as the boundaries.

Well, despite imagining I was infallible, my energy slowly died after about the third day. Although I had made fair inroads into the stack of books, it wasn't enough for the whole area to be completed and I began to panic! I was worn out, exhausted, and my legs and muscles were in sheer agony.

I sought help from my sister in law, and she barely was able to cope to help me. But now, looking back, I dare say she did it out of love and desperation for my state of mind!

Then it came to the last 100 or so to complete the contract I had made. It was a weekend and by Monday I had to sign back in to say the run was complete. Then I would be paid. The task was so big that I just had to ask my husband for a hand. Reluctantly he agreed, and we set off on the Saturday morning with the three children, one was in a stroller and the other two walked. During the first couple of hours things ran smoothly, but for the children, the novelty wore off and they started to whinge that they were thirsty, tired and hungry. We stopped for lunch, after which I expected things would all be okay. Once again, we set off but this time, it didn't go so smoothly!! My nerves were wearing thin, and my temper was ready to boil! First of all, one of my sons had to go the toilet, AGAIN! I argued the point and he started to whinge. So I left the rest of the family to find the toilets in a park some streets away!

He wouldn't walk fast, and complained. I was holding his hand and walking so fast in rage, his little feet were barely touching the pavement! He eventually decided he wasn't going to walk **anymore!** He sat right down on the edge of the lawn. I had also had enough at this stage, and as we reached the lawn of the park near the toilet block, I bent down, grabbed his ankles and dragged him the whole length of the lawned area, while he was crying terrified! People were having their lunch and looking on in shock. I shoved him into the toilet cubicle and screamed at him all the nasty things I could think of, and how inconsiderate he was for doing this to me.

When we made it back to the rest of the family, I was in such a state, that my husband said it was a ridiculous venture, and that I had to finish it off the following week. I disagreed, and said there wasn't that much left to do, and grabbed my trolley full of yellow pages, one of the children, and crossed the road to do the next street. But as I got to the curb, the wheels of the trolley caught the curb and all the books flew all over the road and pavement! This was **it** for me… meltdown began! I looked at them all looking at me, and felt very intimidated and helpless, and was waiting for my husband to come and help. But he didn't, he was beginning to lose it himself, and could not believe what he was seeing. I then screamed. I screamed all kinds of obscenities as though I was a crazy drunk who didn't care about any discretion or courtesy in other peoples neighbourhoods!

This is when enough was enough for my family. My husband took the children, left me where I was and put them into the car and waited for me to come to my senses (if that was at all possible!), but of course, I didn't. I just started howling in a stupor, sat on the pavement and crawled around picking up the books, one by one slowly piling them back onto the trolley. I then got up, still crying inconsolably, pulled the trolley to the trailer, packed everything into the trailer and threw myself at my husband asking him to help me. I really had no idea what was going on.

What had come over me? I went limp and felt totally humiliated at how I had portrayed myself. I hated myself, yet didn't know how to fix it! I think we went home, and on the Monday I had to explain to the yellow pages company that I had fallen ill and couldn't finish the round. I was paid, for only what was delivered. I'm unsure how it all finally transpired!

Weeks after, finally an answer was evident. We saw a documentary about depression. We decided it was time I went to see my doctor. Paralysed with fear and shame, I felt I was unable to go in yet unable to leave. I must have sat there for an age, head in my hands, sobbing inside.

After a long chat, I was diagnosed with what I had already feared and suspected I had... "Manic Depression"! The story from the doctor in Melbourne proved to be **mere rubbish,** and I found out that Manic Depression is **very much hereditary**! I was left with many feelings that day. Firstly, I was upset with the doctor in Melbourne. He could have helped me address these issues long ago. I also felt ashamed, embarrassed, disappointed, **and furious** that I had **my father's genes**. And how I **hated** his dark side! I had sworn I would never be like him. I made it clear to the doctor that I did not want any drugs. I had seen some of my relatives go numb to the point of being unaware of their surroundings and I was going to do my own thing by seeking herbal alternatives.

9. MOVED BY READING

As I look back now and having read many books and articles, this particular author summed up my life for me thus far. *"I've realised there was a particular kind of pain, elation, loneliness and terror involved in this kind of madness. When you're high it's tremendous. The ideas and feelings are fast and frequent. Shyness goes, the right words and gestures are suddenly there, the power to captivate others is felt with certainty. Interest is found in uninteresting people. At times sensuality is persistent and the desire to seduce and be seduced irresistible. Feelings of ease, intensity, power, well-being, financial control, and ecstasy pass through the veins. But, somewhere, this changes. The fast ideas are far too fast, and there are far too many; overwhelming confusion on friends' faces is replaced by fear and concern. Everything previously moving with the grain is now against; you're irritable, angry, frightened, uncontrollable, and trapped totally in the blackest caves of the mind. You never knew those caves were there. It seems it will never end, madness seems to carve its own reality.*

It goes on and on, and finally there are only other's recollections of your behaviour, your bizarre, frenzied, aimless behaviour, for mania has at least some grace in partially erasing memories. What then, after the medications, psychologist, despair, depression, and overdose? There are all those incredible feelings to sort through. Who is being too polite to say what? Who knows what? Who did I do? Why? And most hauntingly, when will it happen again? Then, too, are the bitter reminders; medicine to take, resent, forget, take, resent, and forget, but always to take.

Credit card limits blown and bad credit listed, friendships gone or drained, unsettled marriage. And always, when will it happen again? Which of my feelings are real? Which me is me? Am I the wild, impulsive, chaotic, energetic and crazy one or the shy, withdrawn, desperate, suicidal, doomed and tired one? Probably a bit of both!

My mind scrambled to keep up with itself. Ideas were coming so fast that they intersected one another at every possible angle. There was a neurotic pile up on the highways of my brain, and the more I tried to slow down my thinking the more I became aware that I couldn't. My enthusiasm was going into overdrive as well, but there often was seemed to be a underlying thread of logic in what I was doing."

An Unquiet Mind. Kay Redfield Jamison, Vintage Books. 1995.

10. THE DANGEROUS STOOPS IN THE HIGHS

During this same period of increasingly feverish behaviour, my marriage was falling apart. I had started on a medication which changed a lot of things, the way I was conducting myself and my inner thoughts. Alot was different than ever I had felt before. During this period, I had a brief affair. It wasn't one that included the whole intimate duties like marriage does. But still, the playfulness was total error. We were both married and both also had manic depression. This was the reason for the mess we found ourselves in. I had sympathised with his past, and suddenly I knew I was being sucked into a feeling that I considered was helpful to him. But we all know the dangers of that. It usually does not stop there. I was increasingly restless, irritable, and craved excitement. I found myself rebelling against the very things I most loved about my husband (obviously he had his own human issues, and it usually takes the two of you to be involved when a marriage is on thin ice) But what shone through were his kindness, stability, warmth, protection and love to my mental illness issues. Despite this, I impulsively reached out for a new feeling of love in life.

I felt infinitely worse, more dangerously depressed, guilty of the affair, and in fact felt more dreadful than I had ever felt in my entire life. When the high had passed, I felt dirty and did not know what brought me to stoop so low. I had to figure out how to explain to my husband what I had done. I drove to my parents place and poured out my confession to my mum. I asked for help, and her response was like having an ice block on a hot day! She calmed me down and she gave me those arms as she had so many times before…right around me, and we cried together. She then gave me the advice to go straight to my husband at work and tell him everything I had told her. And I did.

All I can remember was his total silence, sitting by my side, on the left passenger seat of our car. He just stared out the windscreen and said in a nervous, yet monotone voice, *"Is that it? Is that EVERYTHING, I want to know EVERYTHING!"*

I assured him it was. I pleaded and begged for his mercy. I was willing to do anything so that he would not throw me out or tell me to pack my bags when he returned home that day. Of course, because of the man he is, he was not going to throw me out. He said, *"Calm down and we'll sort it all out"*. I felt like I had now jumped into a river of cool water on a boiling day. I could not believe my mums and husbands reactions, the two people I admired the most. After all, I felt like I had let them down and disappointed them so badly, and thought they were going to crush me out of their lives forever. But both were cool, calm, collected and supportive! Was I dreaming? I don't know exactly what I was that day… I knew I was numb all over, sick and **extremely exhausted.** I went home, went to bed and slept, kind of hoping I would wake up and find it had been a terrible nightmare, like many nightmares I had dreamt before! Unfortunately, it was reality, and there was **a lot to repair ahead.**

The first thing was to visit the doctor. My husband had finally figured that the medications may be playing a factor. And off to the quack we went. He had only just prescribed Epilim, the drug I was so frightened of, but reassuringly he said that over the years, they have learnt more about drugs for manic depression, and that he would re-commence me on a low dose. The higher dose had obviously thrown me into a manic high. Basically, Epilim is used for epilepsy, working on the same poles of the brain to help moderate the manic highs and the depressive lows.

While rotating on the planet at the same pace as everyone else, on this medication, I found my spending sprees were over. Mania is not a luxury one can easily afford - it's a devastating illness. Paying for medication, blood tests and counselling is aggravating to the extreme. So after mania, when most depressed, I was given excellent reasons to be even more so!

11. BETRAYAL AND DEPRESSION

I had been mildly manic on many occasions, but they had never been frightening experiences; I was ecstatic at best, confused at worst. As time on the tablets went by, I had learnt to adjust to them quite well. I had developed mechanisms for self-control, to keep down the ring of unusually inappropriate laughter and set severe limits on my irritability. I avoided situations that might otherwise trip or jangle my hypersensitive wiring and I learned to pretend I was paying attention or following a logical point. In fact, my mind was actually chasing rabbits in a thousand different directions. My daily life flowed, but nowhere did this, or my upbringing, my intellect or my character, prepare me for insanity.

The drugs seemed to slow me down, but at the same time we were thrown into turmoil. Firstly, my husband's father had died from the cancer he had been battling with for twelve months. Secondly, within days of his death, we found that one of our closest friends had sexually abused one of our sons over a period of a few months previous. He was only eight at the time.

He, his wife and ourselves had been long-term friends. We (and our children) were close and fond of each other. We had many meals, fun holidays, suppers, picnics and so on together. He had been my husbands mate. He had been part of all our three boys' lives. Now he had betrayed our trust. These events were the beginning of a very bad time not only for me but all of us. Our son too was a victim exposed to "grooming", something which I have previously explained about in earlier chapters. The awful circumstances surrounding the abuse of our son was taken to the law courts and in due course, the perpetrator was convicted.

The entire experience was bad enough but the crippling illness of manic depression exacerbated the impact on all our lives. I am thankful I was on my medication; I had been trying to be sane at best. But something had been building up for months. The "survival mode" of court days were over - I certainly knew something was seriously wrong. There was a definite point when I knew I was insane. Nothing once familiar to me was familiar any longer. I wanted desperately to slow down but couldn't. Nothing helped. My energy level was untouched by anything I did. At one point I was determined that if my mind did not stop racing and begin working normally again, and if I could not get some sleep at last, I would kill myself. I was suicidal. I was causing my loved ones grief, just by my presence! It would be the only kind thing for everyone... they surely would continue normalities after the loss had healed.

We were then left to pick up the pieces of our lives and make amends for the massive amount of quality time we had lost with our children over the past year or so. I basically forgot what beauty in life was all about, and humour or laughter was things I had forgotten how to do!

12. "THAT" FEAR OF LOST FRIENDS – REARS ITS UGLY HEAD

Year by year, as the anniversary of these awful events reared their ugly heads; my condition seemed to worsen around these months. I needed only one more thing to tip me over the edge.

And it was a new friend. I had met her at a mothers' support group for abused children; we became close and depended on one another. After months of lunches and family get-togethers, I decided to tell her about our Christian beliefs and what a positive and wonderful future we believed was ahead of us. I did this in the form of a letter.

But she did not take kindly to my words. And I was shocked when she did not comprehend my religious beliefs. She told me I was crazy and said quite a lot of other hurtful things, then left, never wanting to see me again. This to me was the end of the world. The fear that was in me from a very young age had come to fruition. I could not bare the thought the person I had built a close companionship with was ready and willing to just brush it off as if we had never met before.

I rang her a few times to try and reconcile, and maybe explain the letter I had written was not read in the right way. I expressed that she meant a lot to me, but she did not take me at all seriously, and continued to tell me that she was offended to think that because of our beliefs, our relationship was now different, and that she felt second-rate and that I seemed to think that because I was religious I was better than her. But there was just no solution to the dilemma with her mind set on this understanding of my letter.

The following morning, frustrated and devastated, not a minute of sleep after sobbing the whole night through, I got up feeling delusional. I dropped my children at school and remembered I kept pain killers in the glove box. I remember I still had my pyjamas on. They had become blood-stained from the onset of my period on the way to school. I did not even care, seeing that I was only going to the morgue anyhow. I stopped on the side of the road, sobbing inconsolably, opened the bottle, and with my quivering hands, poured out an unknown amount of strong pain relief pills. I threw them into my mouth, grabbed the bottle of water and swallowed them all in one go. I sat there for a moment, numb and in sheer darkness. I rummaged around for my mobile and rang my husband. I said I was sorry- I just could not stand giving everyone the pain of my existence any longer- I was tired and wanted to go to sleep forever, never to wake up.

I remember him being empathetic yet firm as he asked about the situation into which I had gotten myself. He did not let me hang up and asked where I was. I was drowsy and vaguely recalled the location. I told him that I had planned on driving to my former doctor who had moved to a new practice 30kms away, but gave up hope on the way and overdosed instead. He told me to continue driving there slowly. At this stage, I was like a robot. I was drowsy. I started to panic as I realized that I may have done serious lethal damage this time. I thought the tablets might absorb more quickly as more blood was pumping through my heart and brain. I still did not care at this stage. I kept driving, swerving all over the road and drove slowly as he had instructed me to. In the meantime, he rang the surgery, and they had an ambulance waiting for me.

13. THE $650 RIDE!

I stumbled out of the car, with blood stained flannelette pyjamas. The doctor I wanted to see was the only one I trusted with my life; only he knew my history of depression. Apparently he was busy so I was attended by another one as well as the clinic's nurse. They laid me down, asked a series of questions and checked my vital signs. And in between alternately falling asleep and panicking, a slight realisation dawned on me that I had actually done something quite serious. I was taken to hospital by ambulance to be met there by my husband. Although I was partially asleep while my vital signs were being taken, I remember hearing the nurses and doctor ask my husband about my history of illness and what medication I was taking. I vaguely heard them saying, *"She's very lucky - if she had only taken a couple more, she may have gone into cardiac arrest or a coma"*. But all I had done was seriously lower my blood pressure and made my stomach very irritable. I cannot imagine how my husband was feeling at my side!

I was released much later that night, and remember having to walk out through the emergency room, in front of other patients.

I still wore my blood-stained pyjamas, looked ragged and pale and all I wanted was to go home and have a shower, change my clothes, have something to eat and go back to bed.

The next morning, I realised how close I was to death. I went outside with my cup of tea - the sky seemed bluer, the air smelt fresher and the sun felt warmer. I had chills down my spine thinking "I may not have been standing there that very day! I imagined my lifeless body, on a metal trolley in a fridge, and my family mourning and rushing around doing funeral arrangements, and others trying to console my boys, and yet I was not there to hug them or comfort them - others were doing that job for me! How dare they, that was my job, only I knew them, they were my boys, they only needed me!" While I was deep in this thought, I made sure it was firmly impacted in the corners of my mind.

We went back to my local doctor with a letter from the hospital, suggesting a reassessment of my medication. He changed the type of drug I was on and I was referred to the mental health system for a series of counselling sessions (in my opinion, worthless hours). While in the waiting room with what were evidently "crazy" people, people who visited daily for their injections for who knows what, a gross man was looking at me talking about being Robinson Crusoe and how he lived on his island. He totally freaked me out! There was no way I was coming back after that day. I realised I was on the receiving end of a very thorough psychiatric examination and documentation of my history. I found it unnerving to have to answer the questions, unnerving not to know where it all was going and unnerving to realize how confusing I felt in this position.

I had pages of questions to be answered before I could even begin my counselling. The questions included How many hours of sleep had I been getting? Did I have any problems concentrating? Had I felt pressure to talk constantly? Had I been more energetic than usual? Were other people finding it difficult to keep up with me? Had I been more agitated than usual? Angrier, irritable etc. etc. I did not have the energy to recap all this again. Could not my doctors fax their notes? I was ready to walk right out of the room.

Weeks later the postie delivered the cost of my attempt to "check out of my life". It cost us $650! We did not even have ambulance cover. It is something we do have now though, but not because my next attempt will cost the family less, but just because the realisation of any emergency may be a bit easier on the bank account.

It was a very long time, until I recognized my mind again, and much longer until I trusted it.

14. COMFORT IN OTHER SUFFERERS' STORIES

I recently read an article about a lady who dealt with manic depression and suicide. She made so much sense to me it was like we were having a face-to-face conversation, and I was saying, "Yes, I know exactly what you are saying"!

"Within psychiatric circles, if you kill yourself, you earn the right to be considered a 'successful' suicide. This is a success one can live without. Suicidal depression, I decided in the midst of my indescribably awful, eighteen month bout of it, is God's way of keeping manics in their place. It works. Profound melancholia is a day-in, day-out, night-in, night-out, almost major level of agony. It is a pitiless, unrelenting pain that affords no window of hope, no alternative to a grim and salty existence, and no respite from the cold undercurrents of thought and feeling that dominate the horribly restless nights of despair. There is an assumption, in attaching Puritan concepts such as 'successful' and 'unsuccessful' to the awful, final act of suicide, that those who 'fail' at killing themselves not only are weak, but incompetent, incapable, even of getting their dying quite right. Suicide, however, is almost always an irrational act and seldom is it accompanied by the kind of rigorous intellect that goes with one's better days. It is also often impulsive and not necessarily undertaken in the way one originally planned. I, for example thought I had covered every contingency. I could not stand the pain any longer, could not abide the bone-weary and tiresome person I had become, and felt that I could not continue to be responsible for the turmoil I was inflicting upon my friends and family. In a perverse linking within my mind I thought that, like the pilot whom had seen kill himself to save the

lives of others, I was doing the only fair thing for the people I cared about; it was also the only sensible thing to do for myself. One would put an animal to death for far less suffering!"

An Unquiet Mind. Kay Redfield Jamison, Vintage Books. 1995.

15. DR. REJECTION

A couple of months later, I thought I would do a follow up visit with my doctor, who apparently was busy the day I attempted suicide. I was in a much better place in my mind by now, and wanted to update him on the events since that day. When I was called to his room, I was not greeted with the usual smile. In fact, there was virtually no eye contact at all. Instead he was stern and irritable. He asked what I wanted, and I said I was there to let him know how I was now going.

Much to my surprise, he said that he did not want to treat me any longer! I took a moment and did not think I heard him right. Maybe he was going to retire? So I asked him to clarify what he had said.

He said (as he was closing my file), that I had *"let him down!!!!"*

I started to quiver, knots formed in my stomach and a lump was in my throat as I said, *"Pardon? I what?"*

With his German accent, he repeated, *"We had a deal, and you let me down."*

Now I was totally confused. My body slowly went limp, the fresh and clear mind with which I started the day was now clouded with despair, disbelief and confusion. A DEAL! – what was he on about?!

Could a doctor reject his patient like this? He got up from his chair and opened the door saying, *"All right, thanks, goodbye."*

To this day, I still feel the huge piece of me that was left on his desk! This was a huge trigger for my moods, and once again, I became depressed and again went to a very dark place.

At this point in my life now, looking back, I could not imagine leading a normal life without both taking medication and having the benefits of counselling. However, medication prevented my seductive and disastrous highs, diminished my depression and cleared the wool and webbing from my disordered thinking. It was able to slow me down, keep me from ruining more relationships. It also kept me alive, out of hospital and made therapy possible. Overwhelmingly, I found therapy helped me to heal. It made some sense of the confusion, reined in the terrifying thoughts and feelings, and returned some control, hope and the possibility of learning from my experiences.

16. IT'S ENOUGH TO MAKE YOU PULL YOUR HAIR OUT

During the period of months that I attended the mothers' support group, there was another lady with who I had a very illuminating conversation with about nervous habits. She had openly discussed with us the shameful disorder she had called "trichotillomania". It seemed a mouthful at the time. Being one of the millions of disorders there is in the world, and because we did not know what it was, it did not grab my attention. But as she kept talking, she alerted us to the fact that she did not have much hair on her head, apparently due to the fact that this disorder had totally taken over her life. She continued to say that she compulsively had enjoyment by pulling out her hair strand by strand. She then studied the roots, and sometimes even ate the hair. She had a cropped head because of this, because it made it difficult for her to grasp it.

This raised my eyebrows - I put it in my memory bank to chat to her after the session was over.

I myself had been prone to doing this for many years, but even more so recently during the periods of major stress. When I chatted to her later, she basically said that she also attended another support group for this as well.

I was thankful that I had not had to cut my hair, but I was guilty of very skimpy eyebrows, scarce eyelashes and a small bald patch beside my parted hairline which I would attack.

When I was in deep thought during periods of stress, I would sit and find my spots that I had carefully chosen over my head, pull out the hairs that seemed coarser than the rest, and twang 'em out! But even more, I would study the roots, bite them off and discard the hair. Obviously, this was done in private; I would not just sit with a group of people, or have coffee with my friends and just munch away!

Oh dear… Here was another thing on my profile of "disorders" I remember doing this as far back as high school.

So I went home that afternoon, and searched the Internet for the information. And it all began to make sense.

Here are some of the things I found out.

Symptoms:

Constant tugging, pulling, or twisting of hair

*Increasing sense of tension is present before
the hair pulling*

*Sense of relief, pleasure, or gratification is reported after the hair
pulling*

Hair pulling leads to an uneven appearance

Bare patches or diffuse (all across) loss of hair

*Hair regrowth in the bare spots feels like
stubble*

*Some individuals may develop a bowel obstruction if they eat the hair
they pull out*

Other self-injury behaviours may be present

People suffering from this disorder often deny pulling out their hair

The reason for many mental health specialists defining this disorder as impulse control is that those with this disorder cannot resist the urge to pull their hair. The impulse to pull one's hair is so overpowering that it cannot be controlled. Once the urge has reached those dimensions, there is no way for the person to resist the urge. The result is that bald spots emerge on the scalp. The presence of these bald spots becomes a source of great distress, particularly for teenage girls at a time when they are at the height of concern about their appearance. In fact, it is the impact on appearance and its social consequences which has the greatest impact on social and emotional adjustment of people with this disorder.(Posted by Allan N. Schwartz, LCSW, PhD)

A worthwhile book on the topic written specifically for the public is by Fred, Penzell, PhD titled: *The Hair Pulling Problem: A Complete Guide to Trichotillomania*

(Oxford Universities Press, 2003).

17. TRICHOTILLOMANIA (from Wikipedia)

(TTM), or "trich" as it is commonly known. The name derives from Greek tricho- (hair) plus mania. Is an *impulse control disorder* characterized by the repeated urge to pull out scalp hair, eyelashes, facial hair, nose hair, pubic hair, eyebrows or other body hair, sometimes resulting in noticeable bald patches. Trichotillomania is classified in the *DSM-IV* as an *impulse control disorder*, but there are still questions about how it should be classified. It may seem, at times, to resemble a habit, an addiction, a tic disorder or an obsessive-compulsive disorder. TTM seems to strike most frequently in the pre- or early adolescent years. The typical first-time hair puller is 12 years old, although TTM has affected people as young as one and as old as seventy. It is thought that ninety percent of those with TTM are women, but research is inconclusive and it may simply be the case that men are less likely to seek treatment and can more easily hide their symptoms. A form of TTM that affects very young children appears to occur in males and females at an equal rate and seems to be more benign in nature.

Characteristics: *Individuals with trichotillomania live relatively normal lives; however, they may have bald spots on their head, among their eyelashes, pubic hair, or brows. An additional psychological effect can be low self-esteem, often associated with being shunned by peers and the fear of socializing due to appearance and negative attention they may receive. Some people with TTM wear hats, wigs, eyebrow pencil, or style their hair in an effort to avoid such attention. There seems to be a strong stress-related component. In low-stress environments, some exhibit no symptoms (known as 'pulling') whatsoever. This 'pulling' often resumes upon leaving this environment.*

Many clinicians classify TTM as habit behaviour, in the same family as nail biting (onychophagia) or compulsive skin picking (dermatillomania). These disorders are a cross between mental disorders, such as obsessive compulsive disorder (OCD) because the sight or feel of a body part causes the individual anxiety, and physical disorders such as stereotypic movement disorder because the person performs repetitive movements without being bothered by or completely aware of them. The current classification of trich as an impulse disorder with pyromania, pathological gambling and kleptomania, has been called into question as inadequate and in need of revision. One study showed that individuals with TTM have decreased cerebellar volume. Like people with other OCD-related disorders (for example, body dysmorphic disorder, impulse control disorder, kleptomania, Tourette syndrome), people with TTM have a reduced ability to transport serotonin at the presynaptic level. Anxiety, depression and OCD are more frequently encountered in people with TTM. People with TTM may also eat/chew the roots of the hair that they pull, referred to as trichophagia. In extreme cases this can lead to Rapunzel syndrome, and even death. Some individuals with TTM may feel they are the only person with this problem due to low rates of reportage."

Well, how about that! But I find that being on my antidepressants, the urge to pull out hair is minimal. But I do daily, I still peck a few. Usually I would find myself in the habit whilst driving, and stressing at traffic lights (if only my leg hairs were a bit longer, I would save on beauty waxing costs).

18. LIFE COACH

Once you find the right person to whom pour out your life and trust, counselling is both a sanctuary and a battleground. I did finally find that gentleman; it was the husband of a volunteer at the 'Mood Disorders Association', where support groups were held for others suffering from manic depression. My husband and I joined this Association for a little while. It was evident that to survive, I needed both the pills and the counselling, and he needed support groups and information.

Once I was feeling slightly better, and the 6-8 allocated sessions of counselling were completed, the absolute confidence I felt made it very difficult for me to believe that I even had an illness.

For years after my initial diagnosis I was reluctant to take my prescribed medication. Why was I so unwilling? Why did I have to go through more episodes of mania, followed by long suicidal depressions, before I would take it as prescribed?

Some of my reluctance, no doubt, stemmed from a fundamental denial that I had a real disease. Apparently, this is a common reaction and through my research of manic depression, I have found that these attitudes are commonplace. Moods are in fact, an essential part of the substance of life, shaping ones view of oneself. In my case, I had a horrible sense of loss for who I had been and where I had been, and where I was heading.

My family and friends expected that I would welcome being 'normal', be appreciative of medication and take normal energy and sleep in my stride. But if you're accustomed to only four or five hours of sleep at night, or none at all, it's a very real adjustment to blend into the three-piece suit schedule.

At times, if I was in the middle of a manic sewing or a re-organizing room project, I may have gone two days without any sleep. While comfortable to many, this new routine to which I had been retrained to adjust to by my life coach, I felt life was restricted, less productive and less exciting. When I complain of feeling less lively, energetic or high-spirited, people say, *"Now you're like the rest of us"*, meaning to reassure me that it's OK. But I compare myself with my former self, not with others. Not only that, I tend to compare myself with the best, which I feel I have been, that of course is when I have been mildly manic. When I am my present 'normal' self, I'm far removed from when I have been my liveliest, most productive, most intense, most outgoing and bubbly. In short, for myself, I am a hard act to follow.

Sometimes life coaches come in the form of supportive individuals. It could just be in others who empathise or sympathise. One particular individual is my little sister. She is dear to my heart. Unfortunately though, she too has been exposed to depression. And although we have a large age gap, we have a very close friendship. We are able to judge each others moods quite understandably and know if it is a day for a chat or a day to just let go and basically catch up later (whenever that may be). We do not take offence to it, because we just know! She sent me a mobile text one day which says it all! "God made us sisters, PROZAC made us friends", (or in our case Efexor-XR).

19. MEDS, MEDS, MEDS!

I believe, without doubt, that manic-depressive illness is a medical illness. I also believe that with rare exceptions, it's something that can not go without medication. However, all these beliefs aside, once I felt I was doing quite well after a period of about eight months stability, I still somehow thought that I ought to be able to carry on without drugs. I thought I would be able to do things my own way.

My doctor disagreed. He thought the benefits of medication far outweighed the side-effects such as massive weight gain, lack of libido (or none), poor appetite, drowsiness, vertigo, nausea and insomnia. The issue was not whether the medication was problematic; it was not whether I missed my highs, it was not whether taking medication was consistent with some idealized belief of my family background. The underlying issue was whether or not I would choose to use it irregularly, and thereby ensure a return of my mania and depression. The choice was now painfully clear to me: madness or sanity, life or death.

I came to the conclusion; it was "**a not so fine madness**".

My manias were now recurring more frequently, and increasingly more confusing. My depression was far more suicidal. I have found through researching my illness that few medications are free of side effects and all things considered, taking them is a vast improvement on the brutal and useless alternative treatments - strait jackets, psychiatric wards or hospitals. While anti-convulsant medications now work very effectively and often with less side effects, they are also an extremely effective drug for many people with manic depressive illness.

The right medicines can alleviate the most serious symptoms of bipolar disorders, but even during periods when you are symptom-free, your functionality, your ability to work, maintain relationships and enjoy yourself may be impaired. Lost dreams, broken relationships, ruined careers and the sullen looks of loved ones can weigh heavily on your own emotions. Over time, the pressure can begin to fracture the protective shell of medication, and the vicious cycle begins anew. By attending to all the contributing factors, you can work toward slowing and eventually stopping a whirlpool.

Also, a common trap is to start taking a combination of medications during a period of crisis and then continuing on the same medication regime after the crisis is resolved. As soon as the crisis is no longer an issue, we can visit the doctor to determine the possibility of scaling back or eliminating some of the medication. Most people with bipolar require some medication throughout their lives, but you and your doctor should seize any opportunity to strip away any unnecessary layers of medications.

In these, lets say naïve days when I hated medication, hated myself, hated life, hated living - that was when I most raged. I foggily remember one incident in the kitchen when making my husbands lunch for the day and getting the children ready for school. While preparing their breakfast, I suddenly snapped! I can not quite remember what triggered it, but it could have been something as simple as the children spilling their bowl of cereal on their cleanly laundered clothes. My pent-up emotions had not been released for weeks. Money issues, personality clashes, court hearings (the abuse incident with one of our sons), and a list as long as my arm transformed me into a screaming mess. I fell into a heap. Banging my fists and stabbing the knife into the breakfast bar, I screamed, *"Why, why, why? I don't want this any more. I want to die. I want this to all go away."* I cried and howled so much that I hyperventilated and passed out on the kitchen floor. I woke up to see three small terrified faces staring down at me. Two of my sons were crying and my husband calmly took them into the lounge to watch cartoons. He helped me up, led me to the bathroom, ran me a bath and rang his boss to say he was taking the day off. What happened after that, I am not sure.

20. IT'S NO WONDER I'M CRAZY!

Without some changes in mood, life would be agonizingly boring, and nobody wants that! But what I would love to fix to my brains' speedometer, is a regulator, something that keeps it travelling between 0 and 65kms per hour, and prevents any sudden changes in speed. The regulator would also alert me to just when I need the water topped up or the petrol is just about to run low. And most importantly, when the radiator is about to blow its cap. But obviously, there is not any such thing. And although medications offer great hope, access to the magic pill remains unresolved. Medications work differently for everyone, a godsend to some and a disaster for others. Medications that you find effective in normalizing your moods may cause irritating side effects for others.

I have found there is a frustrating fine line between madness and normality. Just knowing whether my daily experiences and feelings are due to the time of the month, sleep patterns, tablet dosage, external pressures, money budgets, children's problems is a challenge in itself. I have to balance the scales, whether I am having a good or a bad day (usually the bad depressed dark days are the ones that frustrate me - why am I in that state? It's usually the case that I never really know why I am down there!).

But just adding to the equation of confusion **now**, one night I also found out through mere coincidence, as I was on the Web checking the effects of my drugs on the health of my liver - I discovered that VITAMIN DEFICIENCIES are due to the medications I am taking, Humph! WHATEVER NEXT!

As baffled as I was to find this, I could not help myself reading what was unfolding line by line! Was I meant to find this? Yes, I think I was, and I am very happy to pass it on!

Obviously not everyone is on my cocktail, but I am sure if you do your own Google search, you will find your own little helpers through the "alternative medicine" shelf (I must point out here, that I am **not** a doctor and that you must ask your doctor regardless of what 'Dr. Google' says on your screen!).

Anticonvulsant Interactions with Dietary Supplements:

Biotin
Several controlled studies have shown that long-term anticonvulsant treatment decreases blood levels of biotin. In children, a deficiency of biotin can lead to withdrawn behaviour and a delay in mental development. Adults with low biotin levels might experience a loss of appetite, feelings of discomfort or uneasiness, mental depression, or hallucinations. To avoid side effects, individuals taking anticonvulsants should supplement with biotin either alone or as part of a multivitamin.

Calcium

Individuals on long-term multiple anticonvulsant therapy may develop below-normal blood levels of calcium, which may be related to drug-induced <u>vitamin D</u> deficiency.

L-Carnitine

Several controlled and preliminary studies showed that multiple drug therapy for <u>seizures</u> results in dramatic reductions in blood carnitine levels. Another small study revealed that children taking valproic acid experienced less fatigue and excessive sleepiness following L-carnitine supplementation. Despite the lack of well-controlled studies, individuals who are taking anticonvulsants and experiencing side effects might benefit from supplementing with L-carnitine.

Folic acid

Several studies have shown that multiple anticonvulsant therapy reduces blood levels of folic acid and dramatically increases <u>homocystine</u> levels. Homocystine, a potential marker for folic acid deficiency, is a compound used experimentally to induce seizures and is associated with <u>atherosclerosis</u>. Carbamazepine alone has also been shown to reduce blood levels of folic acid. One well-controlled study showed that adding folic acid to multiple anticonvulsant therapy resulted in reduced seizure frequency. Despite the apparent beneficial effects, some studies have indicated that as little as 0.8 mg of folic acid taken daily can increase the frequency and/or severity of seizures. However, a recent controlled study showed that both healthy and epileptic women taking less than 1 mg of folic acid per day had no increased risk for seizures. Until more is known about the risks and benefits of folic acid, individuals taking multiple anticonvulsant drugs should consult with their healthcare practitioner before supplementing with folic acid.

Vitamin A

One controlled study showed that taking multiple anticonvulsant drugs results in dramatic changes in the way the body utilizes vitamin A.

Vitamin B6

One controlled study revealed that taking anticonvulsant drugs dramatically reduces blood levels of vitamin B6. A nutritional deficiency of vitamin B6 can lead to an increase in homocystine blood levels, which has been associated with atherosclerosis. Vitamin B6 deficiency is also associated with symptoms such as dizziness, fatigue, mental depression, and seizures. On the other hand, supplementation with large amounts of vitamin B6 (80–200 mg per day) has been reported to reduce blood levels of some anticonvulsant drugs, which could theoretically trigger seizures.

People taking multiple anticonvulsant drugs should discuss with their doctor whether supplementing with vitamin B6 is advisable.

Vitamin B12

Anaemia is an uncommon side effect experienced by people taking anticonvulsant drugs. Though many researches believe that low blood levels of <u>folic acid</u> are involved, the effects might be caused by a vitamin B12 deficiency. Deficiencies of folic acid and vitamin B12 can lead to nerve and mental problems. One study revealed that individuals on long-term anticonvulsant therapy, despite having no laboratory signs of anaemia, had dramatically lower levels of vitamin B12 in their cerebrospinal fluid (the fluid that bathes the brain) when compared with people who were not taking seizure medications. Improvement in mental status and nerve function was observed in a majority of symptomatic individuals after taking 30 mcg of vitamin B12 daily for a few days. Another study found that long-term anticonvulsant therapy had no effect on blood levels of vitamin B12. The results of these two studies indicate that people taking anticonvulsant drugs might experience side effects of vitamin B12 deficiency, and that the deficiency is not easily detected by the usual blood tests. Therefore, individuals taking anticonvulsant drugs for several months or years might prevent nerve and mental problems by supplementing with vitamin B12.

Vitamin D

Though research results vary, long-term use of anticonvulsant drugs appears to interfere with vitamin D activity, which might lead to softening of bones (osteomalacia). One study showed that blood levels of vitamin D in males taking anticonvulsants were lower than those found in men who were not taking seizure medication. In a controlled study, bone strength improved in children taking anticonvulsant drugs who were supplemented with the activated form of vitamin D and 500 mg per day of calcium for nine months. Some research suggests that differences in exposure to sunlight—which normally increases blood levels of vitamin D—might explain why some studies have failed to find a beneficial effect of vitamin D supplementation. In one controlled study, blood vitamin D levels in children taking anticonvulsants were dramatically lower in winter months than in summer months. Another study of 450 people in Florida taking anticonvulsants found that few had drug-induced bone disease. Consequently, people taking anticonvulsant drugs who do not receive adequate sunlight should supplement with 400 IU of vitamin D each day to help prevent osteomalacia.

Vitamin E

Two studies showed that individuals taking phenytoin and Phenobarbital had lower blood vitamin E levels than those who received no treatment for seizures. Though the consequences of lower blood levels of vitamin E are unknown, people taking multiple anticonvulsant drugs should probably supplement with 100 to 200 IU of vitamin E daily to prevent a deficiency.

The information presented in *Healthnotes* is for informational purposes only. It is based on scientific studies (human, animal, or *in vitro*), clinical experience, or traditional usage as cited in each article. The results reported may not necessarily occur in all individuals. For many of the conditions discussed, treatment with prescription or over-the-counter medication is also available. Consult your doctor, practitioner, and/or pharmacist for any health problem and before using any supplements or before making any changes in prescribed medications. The "reviews" listed for any medical condition, prescription drug, condition or symptom is provided specifically from eVitamins and is not associated with *Healthnotes*. (Healthnotes, Inc.)

21. FEEL LIKE FISHING?!

Other than the fact I really do like fishing, this is not about the reel, bait and hook type!

Studies have shown that in countries such as Finland and Iceland, where fish is a huge part of the national diet, the rates of depression are lower than in the USA and other parts of Europe. What the scientists discovered was that Omega-3 fatty acids –

essential fatty acids found in fish and other foods show promise in preventing heart disease and in treating depression and auto-immune diseases. But obviously there is no replacement for medications such as mood stabilizer or antidepressants!

22. DEDICATION, NURTURE AND LOVE

When I am seriously irritable, agitated or perturbed, my husband sometimes has a gentling and calming effect on me. Another part of him is charming and funny; he does try to help me see the brighter side of a dull moment. This sometimes works but sometimes does not. Sometimes it is just basically aggravating. But he nursed me through the most awful days of my life and to him only (with my psychologist, family and God) I owe my life.

My mother also was (and still is) wonderful. She would answer the phone whatever the hour of the day or night. Sometimes, in the middle of the night during a manic high, I would ring just to talk to her because it was so quiet in the house while I was sewing or doing crafts, and I needed to chat. She would tell me to wait a minute while she fetched her dressing gown. Then she would take the phone to another room to avoid waking dad. She would chat to me for hours until I was totally exhausted and ready to go to bed in the wee hours of the morning. On the other hand, I would ring her on the not-so-high times. With suicidal thoughts, I would be lying in bed crying to myself. I expressed thoughts that my husband had heard too many times before. He had the same answer and comforting cuddles for me, but I would just want to ring my mum and let her listen to all my woes.

I had fears and lacked confidence in the mothering of my children. I also did not want them to grow up watching me behave in such distressing ways, as I had experienced with my own father. This is the mother I will love forever. She has been like a gentle mother cat that picks up a straying kitten by the nape of its neck. She kept her marvellously maternal eyes wide-open and if I wandered too far away, she brought me back into emotional security and protection. For each terrible storm that came my way, my mother, her love and her strong sense of values, provided me with powerful, sustaining and influential words. I owe her so many hours, which in a lifetime I will never be able to provide. I hope she knows it, and feels that she is the best mother I could ever have in the whole world.

23. LOOKING THROUGH THE WINDOW OF RAGE

These were the feelings of Kay Redfield Jamison that made me feel like my foot fitted into her shoe exactly, the heel to the toe! *"The complexities of what we are given in life are vast and beyond comprehension. By way of temperament, my lot was as if my father had given me an impossibly wild, dark, and unbroken horse, a horse without a name, a horse with no experience of a bit between its teeth. My mother taught me to be gentle with it; she gave me the discipline to love and break it."*

My mania and depression both had violent sides to them. But being a woman, it is somehow more unacceptable than if I were a man. Being wildly out of control, physically aggressive, screaming insanely at the top of my lungs, running frantically without purpose or limit, or impulsively plotting to leap from cars is frightening to others and unspeakably terrifying to oneself. In my blind manic rages, I have done all of these things at one time or another, and some of them repeatedly. I remain acutely and painfully aware of how difficult it is to control or understand such behaviours, much less be able to explain them to others. In my psychotic, seizure-like attacks, my black manias, I have destroyed things I cherish, pushed people I love to the utter edge and survived to think I could never recover from the shame. Among some of these awful times I have been physically restrained against my will by my husband's terrible brute force. I do not know how I recovered from these things which necessitated such actions, any more than I know how or why my relationships with friends and my husband have survived the grinding wear and tear of such dark, fierce and damaging energies. The aftermath of such violence, like the aftermath of a suicide attempt, is deeply bruising to all concerned.

After my suicide attempt, I had to reconcile the image of myself as a young girl, with that of a dreary, pained woman. The first is filled with enthusiasm, high hopes, great expectations, enormous energy and dreams of love and life. The second is one who desperately wished only for death and took an almost lethal dose of pain killers in order to accomplish it!!! After each of my violent episodes, I had to try and reconcile my view of myself as a reasonable, quietly-spoken and highly-disciplined person, one at least generally sensitive to the moods and feelings of others, with an enraged, utterly insane and abusive woman who lost access to all control or reason.

Stress has a bad reputation but it is not always harmful. Negative stress may fill you with overwhelming anxiety and anger; spending too many hours at a job you hate can make you angry and bitter. Positive events on the other hand such as getting a new house or going on a camping trip can stir up your emotions and nervous system just as much as negative ones, and the brain and body perceive them as stressful, even if you are happy. Anything that gets your adrenalin going, good or bad, is a potential trigger for a mood episode. The major changes from the norm are inconceivable and frightening. For instance –

Camping. To even just start to comment about such an idea for the following year, I would go stiff inside, thinking where the camping gear was located in the shed, that the gas bottles needed filling, how many gas bottles would be needed, what condition the tent was in, were all the poles put back last time we used it, what food arrangements I would have to organize, who we were camping near, what bathroom facilities would be available.

Now if you were going to plan a trip, these may seem very normal considerations, but multiply the speed of thoughts by 100, and triple the heart rate too so that your thought process is so totally exhausting that you need to have a nap, and then to wake up hoping that no-one really wants to go away after all.

There are discrepancies between what one is, what one is brought up to believe, is the right way of behaving toward others, and what actually happens during these awful black manias or mixed states. They are absolutely disturbing beyond description, particularly when a woman is brought up in a highly conservative and traditional world. They seem a very long way from my mother's grace and gentleness.

24. WHAT IS TOLERABLE OR ACCEPTABLE?

For the most important formative years of my life, I was brought up in a strait-laced world, taught to be thoughtful for others, circumspect, and restrained in my actions. We went to worship every Sunday and Bible study class every Wednesday. In conversation with people who were not even related to me, all my sentences began with Aunty or Uncle, which was considered a matter of respect to my elders. The independence encouraged by my parents had been of a rational and socially orderly nature. Then suddenly, as an adult, I was unpredictably and uncontrollably irrational and destructive! This was not something that could be overcome by practising decorum. God was clearly nowhere to be found. Uncontrollable anger and violence were dreadfully and irreconcilably distant from my civilized and predictable world.

Depression somehow is much more in line with societies ideas of what women are all about: passive, sensitive, hopeless, helpless, stricken, dependent, confused, rather tiresome, and with limited aspirations. Manic states on the other hand, seem to be more the attributes of men, restless, fiery, aggressive, volatile, energetic, risk-takers, flamboyant, imaginative and impatient. Under such circumstances, anger and irritability in men seems to be more tolerated and understandable.

Fortunately, my friends were either a bit loopy themselves, or remarkably tolerant of the chaos that lay at the basic heart of my emotional existence.

One friend, to whom I mainly refer, would laugh at that very comment. We have shared twenty years of love and experiences. Many late night chats, tears and giggles. All of which have been the mainstay of my existence today. She is reliable and supportive. An SMS message she sent me one day sums up our friendship. This particular occasion I was waiting in a doctor's surgery; the wait had been a long one (as usual), so I messaged her to let her know that I was at the doctor's to re-assess my medications **yet** again. She wrote, *"IT'S A GOOD JOB I LOVE YOU ANY WHICH WAY!"*. To sum her up, she is the woman that brings tears to my eyes while making me smile at the same time!

25. COMING TO TERMS

Mental exhaustion had taken a long, terrible toll, but strangely, it was only when I was feeling well, energetic, and high-spirited that I had any true sense of the toll taken. My moods still shift often and abruptly enough to afford me occasional intoxicating, mind-on-the-edge experiences. The high-flying manias come with assured purpose, and free-flowing cascades of ideas. But when the black tiredness inevitably follows, I would be subdued by the recognition that I had a bad disease, one that could destroy all pleasure and hope and competence. I covet the day-to-day steadiness that most of my friends and family seem to enjoy. I also appreciate how draining and preoccupied I have become just keeping my mind bobbing above water.

It is true that much gets done during the days and weeks of high flying, but it is also true that newly-generated projects and commitments are made, which then have to be completed during the greyer times. I constantly chase the tail of my own brain. But also the body takes its toll with such unnatural energies. Your joints ache, muscles feel heavy and lazy.

The very skin all over the body is sore to touch. Your eyes feel like they are bulging, your scalp feels tight and highly sensitive. Due to being too pre-occupied, not enough fluids (water) are consumed. Your tongue is so dry it clings to the roof of your mouth and seems double its size. Your throat and glands are hot and swollen (as it seems). Eventually the mania dissipates and you are left thinking you are experiencing symptoms of a major illness. Panic and paranoia set in, doctor's appointments are made, and specialists are booked. I ask for numerous tests to be run. And only after all avenues are exhausted do I feel I can move on with freedom from the paranoid thought that I was dying.

Identifying distorted thinking is a tricky thing. Distorted thoughts commonly cloud perception and spark an irrational internal dialogue that can spiral your mood down into depression or up into mania. Thinking that any endeavour will lead to failure, for example, can produce a self-defeating domino effect that results in hopelessness and despair. On the other side, thinking that any endeavour will lead to success, no matter what, can inspire endless optimism. Through cognitive therapy, you can identify the distorted thoughts and patterns that permeate the mind.

Basically, I am deeply sceptical that anyone without this illness can truly understand it. And ultimately, it is probably unreasonable to expect the kind of acceptance and understanding of it that one so desperately desires. It is not an illness that lends itself to easy empathy. Restless or frayed moods that turn to anger or violence - they can seem deliberate and frightening. And it is at these times, impossible for me to convey my desperation and pain; afterward, it is harder still to recover from the damaging acts and dreadful words. These terrible black manias, with their agitated, ferocious and savage sides are understandably difficult for friends, family and loved ones to understand and almost as difficult for me to explain.

No amount of love can cure madness or lighten one's dark moods. But it can help, it can make the pain more tolerable. And always, you are beholden to medication that may or may not work and may or may not be bearable. Madness on the other hand, most certainly can and often does kill love through its distrust, unrelenting negativity, discontent, erratic behaviour and especially, through its savage moods. The sadder, sleepier, slower and less volatile depressions are better understood and more easily taken in stride. Experience and love over much time, have taught me and my closest companion (my husband), a great deal about dealing with manic-depressive illness. I occasionally laugh and think to myself that his calming demeanour and yet sarcastic humour is worth to me, three hundred milligrams of my medication a day. And it's probably true! Sometimes, in the midst of one of my dreadful destructive upheavals, I feel his quietness nearby and am reminded that although he may be lacking the words to help, he will just sit nearby, as if to say, "I am here if you need me - when you are ready." So if love is not the cure, it certainly can act as a very strong medicine.

26. CLINICAL TERMINOLOGIES

I have used the term "manic-depression" but in actual fact I was diagnosed with "bi-polar disorder". Recently I read some literature about the differences (if any) and why there are two different terms:

"In the language that is used to discuss and describe mental illness, many different things, descriptiveness, clinical precision, and stigma-intersect to create confusion, misunderstanding and a gradual bleaching out of the traditional words and phrases. It is no longer clear what place words such as "mad", "daft", "crazy", or "cracked" should have in a society increasingly sensitive to the feelings and rights of those who are mentally ill. Should, for example, expressive, often humorous, language-phrases such as "taking the fast trip to Squirrel City" being a "few apples short of a basket", "off the planet", "around the bend", "a brick short of a pallet"- "fruitcake", "nut", "wacko", "loon", be held hostage to the fads and fashions of "correct" or "acceptable" language? Using these words, it was felt, would "carry on a lack of self esteem, and self-stigmatization" to certain individuals. No doubt, allowing such language to go unchecked or uncorrected leads not only to personal

pain, but contributes both directly and indirectly to discrimination in jobs, insurance and society at large. On the other hand, the assumption that rigidly rejects words and phrases that have existed for centuries will have much impact on public attitudes is rather dubious. It gives an illusion of easy answers to impossibly difficult situations and ignores the powerful role of wit and positive agents of self-notion and social change. Clearly there is a need for freedom, diversity, wit and directness of language about abnormal mental states and behaviour. Just as clearly, there is a profound need for a change in public perception about mental illness. The issue, of course, is one of context and emphasis. Science, for example requires highly precise language. Too frequently, the fears and misunderstandings of the public, the needs of science, the inanities of popularized psychology, and the goals of mental health advocacy get mixed together in a diverse confusion.

One of the best cases is the current confusion of the use of the increasingly popular term "Bipolar disorder" – now firmly entrenched in the book "Diagnostic and Statistical Manual" (DSM-IV), the authoritative diagnostic system published by the American Psychiatric Association-instead of the historic term "Manic-depressive illness" . As a person and patient, however, I find the word "Bipolar" strangely and powerfully offensive: it seems to me to obscure and minimise the illness it is supposed to represent the description "manic-depressive," on the other hand, seems to capture both the nature and the seriousness of the disease I have, rather than attempting to paper over the reality of the condition.

Most clinicians and many patients feel that "bipolar disorder" is less stigmatizing than "manic-depressive illness". Perhaps so, but perhaps not. Certainly, patients who have suffered from the illness should have *the right to choose whichever term they feel more comfortable with. But the two questions arise: Is the term "bipolar" really a medically accurate one and does changing the name of a condition actually lead to a greater acceptance of it? The answer to the first question, which concerns accuracy, is that "bipolar" is accurate in the sense that is indicates an individual has suffered from both mania (and mild forms of mania) and depression alone. But splitting mood disorders into bipolar and unipolar categories presupposes a distinction between depression and manic-depressive illness-both clinically and etiologically – that is not always clear, nor supported by science. Likewise it perpetuates the notion that depression exists rather tidily segregated on its own pole, while mania clusters off neatly and discreetly on another. This polarization of two clinical states flies in the face of everything that we know about the fluctuating nature of manic and depressive states, conditions that are common, extremely important clinically, and lit at the heart of many of the critical theoretical issues underlying this particular disease."*

An Unquiet Mind. Kay Redfield Jamison, Vintage Books. 1995.

27. CLARIFYING THE LABEL

(from *"Bipolar Disorder for Dummies"* Candida Fink, MD. Joe Kraynak)

"If you're like most people, you shun labels – especially labels that carry negative connotations, such as BIPOLAR. Used in a sentence, such as "Pat is bipolar," the label seems even more insensitive. It not only stigmatizes Pat, but also reduces her to the illness itself. If Pat had

cancer, nobody would say, "Pat is cancer," but people often play fast and loose with the term "bipolar".

You're physician or psychiatrist doesn't use the label "bipolar disorder" to label you or minimise your worth as a human being. The label provides a convenient way to refer to your condition that requires treatment. It helps all the people involved in your treatment plan to quickly recognize the disease that afflicts you and to provide the appropriate medications and therapy."

In actual fact I even fell into this trap for quite some time. I would see myself as one person with a filthy cloak hanging off my shoulders that had a brand name tag, "Made by Bipolar".

This cloak would be with me most times, and sometimes I was able to take it off to give it a wash. I was happy when I could wash it, but it always went straight back on me, and very quickly it would become soiled and dirty again.

I was very conscious that everyone noticed. It was part of me. I just could not shrug it off. I would make it obvious to people that the cloak was me. I knew it was because the doctor had told me so. Sometimes I would have a complex about how I came across to people. I was very insecure, and still am. In some ways, I maybe was too overbearing, too over-excitable, or too blunt and rude.

There was an occasion I recall, that the receptionist at my sons school seemed always to have the least to say to me when I was at the desk needing information or having a payment to make.

But I could see she was very cheerful to the other parents. I took note of this for around five months and finally I convinced myself that I must have aggravated or upset her in some way or other. So I took it on myself to write her a letter. I don't remember exactly the wording but it went something along the lines of:

"Dear Julie,

I feel like I need to write to you and apologize for anything I have done to upset you. I seem to feel that you are very blunt with me when I need something, and yet you are cheerful to other people. I know that your job is very demanding, and I wouldn't replace your position any time, but I have waited for some time and watched how we communicate and feel I just have to sort it out. I have had a shocking past 12 months, and I may also have come across rather rude and grumpy at times. I have bipolar disorder, and this has been very hard for me to come to grips with. Sometimes I don't even know if I have upset people, that's why I need to clarify with you if I have done anything which could have offended you at any time.

I hope you understand, and if you would like to chat about this you can call me on my contact phone no.

Regards Adele".

I handed this letter to her the next morning with a small packet of chocolates. She seemed taken aback at the time, obviously not knowing what occasion this may be for.

I received a phone call about three days later. She said that of course she did not have anything against me, and that I had never upset her either. She just was so busy in her new position, and that things just stress her out rather quickly. She was sorry to hear I had been suffering from bipolar disorder, and that she would never have guessed.

Well, how stupid I felt then. I burst into tears with the relief of the five months of building up the thoughts, fears and stress of the whole matter.

This is not the only time that I felt that I was BIPOLAR, and not ME. I have now concluded that I am not bipolar, and bipolar is not me. And the massive amounts of counselling and research have helped me put this to rest – FINALLY! Candida Fink's book *"Bipolar Disorder for Dummies"* at last clarified the issue for me. Now I just want to educate family, friends and any others that need to differentiate the two!

28. RESTRUCTURING THOUGHTS AND BEHAVIOURS

So I had decided enough was enough. My mind was sending me round the bend. I was tired through exhaustive analysis and replaying scenarios over and over again, month after month. So out came the books again. Again I found more fantastic matter in *"Bipolar Disorder for Dummies"*:

"Thought precipitates action, inaction. If you don't think you can ever have a fulfilling relationship, you may not have the motivation to try. If you believe you're entitled to have everything you want, despite the cost, you may not hesitate to act, no matter how high the risk. The ultimate goal of Cognitive Behavioural Therapy is to change your behavioural responses from self-defeating and negative to productive and realistic. This change creates positive experiences that support positive moods.

Cognitive Behavioural Therapy goes beyond thought to behaviour, or action. In the case of debilitating depression, Cognitive Behavioural Therapy attempts to identify the restrictive thought, question its validity, reveal other possibilities and encourage you to take action.

Approaches vary, depending on the distortion and how it works in a particular instance. A qualified therapist can recommend several techniques for identifying and ridding your mind of distorted thoughts."

29. TOCK-TICK

The world has a rhythm to it: the tick-tock of the clock, sunrise-sunset, the phases of the moon, the outgoing tide and flow of tides, the work week, seasonal shifts, paydays, TV show times.

And you subconsciously move to the rhythms around you. As long as they remain relatively in tune with healthy routines, you do just fine. But when an event throws off your natural rhythm, your moods can shift out of their normal orbit.

Manic depressive sufferers commonly find solace in a structured routine. Routine calms. It orders the chaos. It removes unpleasant surprises. It simplifies planning. And it helps you get a good nights sleep, night after night, because sleep deprivations can trigger mania. But unfortunately, keeping a routine can be a joke, especially when you are a little manic, which is when you most need the calming effects of routines.

There is a challenge - try to complete a weekly schedule, examine it for the most dramatic variations, then draw up a new one with less variations. Do not make drastic changes that you can not possibly keep. Go slowly. Adjustments can be done at a later stage. Formulating goals and helping yourself slowly accept realistic changes assists in preventing triggers for moods.

But when you finally feel you are in tune with the universe, you get a one-two punch! Christmas... New Year! And in a matter of days, scheduling changes, crowded shopping centres, and dysfunctional relations trash your well-tuned biological clock! And soon you don't hear the constant pattern of its rhythm. But you hear a *tock-tick, tock-tock-tick! and* so on.

The best thing to do is to plan for these times so you anticipate such events and curb the effects of any unforseen incidents. By pre-planning holidays, weekends, birthdays and other bigger celebrations, you do not leave yourself open to unrestrained spontaneity, which may lead to manic impulsivity.

30. HEREDITARY GENEALOGY

Oddly enough, it had never occurred to me to not have children because I had this manic-depressive illness. Being naïve to the fact that it's hereditary, I fell pregnant in ignorance of the possible consequences. The doctor in Melbourne could have been very much more helpful by providing relevant information in this regard!

Even in my blackest depressions, I have never regretted having been born. It's true that I had wanted to die, but that is peculiarly different from regret at being born. I have been overwhelmingly glad and grateful for life and could not imagine not wanting to pass on life to someone else. All things considered, I have had a marvellous though turbulent and occasionally awful existence. Of course, I have had serious concerns. How could I not? Would I, for example, be able to take care of my children properly? What would happen to them when I became severely depressed? Much more frightening still, what would happen to them if I became manic, if my judgment became impaired, if I became violent or uncontrollable? How would it be watching my own children struggle with depression, hopelessness, despair, or insanity if they themselves became ill? Would I watch them too hawkishly for symptoms or mistake their normal reactions to life as signs of illness? All of these are things that cross my mind, but never have I regretted having them. I have quite often said that those with manic depression should not do two things... 1. Get Married and 2. Have children. These are two very demanding responsibilities for even a so-called normal individual. In fact, I believe it is one of the factors preventing complete recovery from the illness or at least stability.

Stress is an enormous factor in the high and low swings. And if you can just live a single, stable and structured life style, with the love and support of friends and family, I believe it is very possible to manage, or be cured from it. But this is mere assumption on my behalf and I have not researched or seen any literature supporting that.

What I have read is the thought and theory. If laboratories can track the genes in unborn foetuses, is it right to let the prospective parents choose to abort foetuses that carry the genes for manic-depressive illness, even though it is treatable?

One article states, *"Do we risk making the world a blander, more homogenized place if we get rid of the genes for manic-depressive illness. An admittedly impossibly complicated scientific problem? What are the risks to the risk takers, those restless individuals who join with others in society to propel the arts, business, politics, and science? Are manic-depressives, like spotted owls and clouded leopards, in danger of becoming an "endangered species"?*

These are very difficult ethical issues, particularly because manic-depressive illness can confer advantages on both the individual and society. The disease, in both its severe and less severe forms, appears to convey its advantages not only through its relationship to the artistic temperament and imagination, but through its influence on many eminent scientists, as well as business, religious, military, and political leaders. Subtler effects- such as those on personality, thinking style, and energy- are also involved because it is a common illness with a wide range of temperamental, behavioural, and cognitive expression. The situation is yet further complicated by the fact that additional genetic, biochemical, and environmental factors (such as exposure to prolonged or significant changes in light, pronounced sleep reduction, childbirth, drug and alcohol use) may be at least in part responsible for both the illness and the cognitive and temperamental characteristics associated with great achievement. These scientific and ethical issues are real ones; fortunately, they are being actively considered by the federal Governments Genome Project and other groups of scientists and ethicists. But they are immensely troubling problems and will remain so for many years."

An Unquiet Mind. Kay Redfield Jamison, Vintage Books. 1995

31. WHERE IN THE BRAIN DOES BIPOLAR FORM?

(from *"Bipolar Disorder for Dummies"* Candida Fink, MD. Joe Kraynak)

Pinpointing the location of bipolar disorder in your brain is almost as difficult as finding affordable health insurance. Your brain consists of about 100 billion cells of two different types: neurons and glial cells. Neurons form the telecommunications network in the brain, enabling the cells to communicate with one another and carry signals back and forth between your brain and the rest of your body. Glial cells act as the brain's caretaker - ensuring that the neurons have the chemicals and nutrients they need to function, repairing damaged brain cells, and keeping infection at bay.

Within the cerebrum, the brain is further divided. The cerebrum cortex is the outermost layer of the brain, commonly referred to as the grey matter. Below that layer are bundles of long nerve fibres called white matter that carry information between parts of the brain. Deep in the brain are subcortical areas, such as the limbic system, including the amygdala, hippocampus, and cingulate gyrus.

These areas are involved in emotional control, drive the motivation, fear responses, and memory. Many brain function studies reveal that these areas of the brain function differently in people with bipolar disorder or depression compared to those without these illnesses. The brain science behind bipolar disorder is just beginning to mature. The concept of a simple chemical imbalance, although appealing, isn't quite accurate. Bipolar disorder more likely is the result of various blips in the brain circuitry that foul up the operations of various departments and scramble communications between departments.

Although various areas of the brain are suspected conspirators in producing bipolar symptoms, doctors can not restructure the brain to repair the abnormalities. Instead, they choose the less intrusive option of adjusting the way the brain transfers signals via its neurotransmitters.

When your brain functions properly, it reacts appropriately to stimulation. Someone cuts you off in traffic; you angrily honk your horn. You win a prize on the radio; you jump for joy.
When your brain malfunctions, it may overreact inappropriately. You may feel depressed at parties or excited when your sister-in-law shows photos of her new kitchen.

When your moods are out of sync with reality, your brain's physiology or chemistry may be off balance. A psychiatrist fondly referred to by many with bipolar disorder as a p-doc, helps adjust the biochemistry or you brain to enable it to respond appropriately. This does not cure your bipolar disorder, but it helps regulate your moods so you can function and begin to deal with real-life issues that may trigger your mood swings.

32. THROUGH MY CHILDREN'S EYES

Manic depression has swept a broad path across our lives. The untroubled grace of early mania inevitably deteriorated into days, or weeks of fierce and relentless incoherence.

The children were witnesses to the rages, tears, panic attacks. Smashed dishes, slammed doors, neglected animals, unwatered plants, meal-less meals, an untidy home, (as if someone had broken in during the day and trashed the place while I was asleep). Washing duties had been neglected so no clothes to wear. I did not bathe or change mine or the children's clothes during these episodes. I didn't eat or sleep much. The boys would have been placed in front of the TV watching cartoon episodes that ran all day. The pantry and fridge was used like a smorgasbord for the day. I sustained myself with chocolate and coffee, usually in enormous quantities.

Friends, family and of course I, were horrified, helpless, embarrassed. Yet, on the other hand, I was living in the murky realm of the underworld gods. With them at my back, I staggered righteously through the darkness, laying waste to everything and everybody in sight. The children were probably most privy to my undignified behaviours. They were the ones reliant on me, and would think no mother would be any different. I was the only one they ever knew as their carer.

I can only imagine the awkwardness I have caused them on many an occasion. Their little pitter-patters towards my dark room would often result either in me screaming at them or just lying in my bed like a dead stiff.

So often I would feel little fingers sweep through my hair. Or little warm soft lips kiss mine, even a soft whisper, while rubbing my back saying they loved me. I would often wake up, only to go to the toilet, and find that one or two of them had brought their pillows into my room and lay down either on the floor or on the bed next to me. They would have their favourite toy, book or Lego by their side, which said to me that they must have been there for a while, perhaps waiting to see some life in me. This creates a knot in my stomach, just as I write this, coming to the realisation of the many dark days I lay lifeless and incoherent to what the world around me was doing.

As they have grown older, I would wake to a cold cup of coffee next to me, or even a little note or picture with encouraging words that reminded me that they loved me. I have been blessed with the way the children have just managed on their own. They have never got up to major mischief considering the numerous opportunities that have presented themselves.

I have to look to the heavens though, and realize that our heavenly Father was looking down through our roof tiles, and placed angels in the rooms where my children were sitting, caring for them during the very bleak times when their dad was not able to be around, while he was hard at work.

I am very proud of our boys. I will always remember them for their honourable trustworthiness and love to me, their mum.

33. TO THOSE ON THE OTHER SIDE

Imagine yourself cruising down the highway at a comfortable speed of 75 km per hour, when your cruise control goes berserk. The speedometer climbs to 95 and then 110 … you hit the button to cancel…tap the brakes…nothing slows you down. .120…your car is shaking and weaving…130…people are honking…145 …police are chasing you…150…your spouse is yelling and calling you CRAZY, and pleading for you to SLOW DOWN…185…200..

Or perhaps imagine the opposite: You are driving through town, at the 40 km per hour speed limit, nobody in front of you, and your car can only go 10km per hour. You're practically pushing the accelerator through the floor, but you can only get it up to 15, 20km per hour maximum …downhill!!! Your neighbours are honking, passing you on the right - on bicycle - giving you dirty looks and other gestures of annoyance.

Well, when you have manic-depression, your brains accelerator is stuck. At full speed, it launches into a manic episode. In slow gear, it grinds you down into a deep depression.

If this were your heart, somebody would call the ambulance. Doctors and nurses would flock to your bedside, loved ones would fly in from other states, and you would get flowers and fruit baskets. But when your brain is stuck in park or overdrive, people just think you are lazy, you have snapped, or you are too weak to deal with life. Instead of flowers and fruit baskets, you get a prescription, bunch of admission papers to fill out, and if you are not married to the type of man I am – the divorce papers. The good news is that the mind mechanics – psychiatrists, psychologists, and therapists – have tool boxes packed with medications and therapies that can repair your brains accelerator.

34. WHO AM I, WHO SHOULD I BE?

There is no easy way to tell other people that you have manic-depressive illness, if there is, I have not found it. So despite the fact that most people have been very understanding of my condition, some remarkably so, I remain haunted by those occasions when the response was unkind, condescending, or lacking in even a semblance of empathy.

I recall the time when the doctor told me I had 'let him down'. I also recall a very close friend who grew up with me and seemed to disbelieve there was such a thing. I felt betrayed, deeply embarrassed and utterly exposed. Otherwise of course, her care knew no bounds. I should have told her not to worry, that manic-depression was not contagious. Although she could have benefited from a bit of mania, given her rather dreary, obsessive and humourless view of the world.

I have been particularly concerned with my clients. If they knew of my manic-depressive illness, would that affect their perception of who I am and what I do? There is a thin line between what's considered zany and what is thought to be "inappropriate," a ghastly but damning word. Only a sliver of a gap exists between being thought intense, or a bit volatile, and being dismissed as "unstable". And for whatever reasons of personal vanity, I dread the fact that my suicide attempt and depressions will be seen by some as acts of weakness or as "neurotic". Somehow, I do not mind being considered as intermittently psychotic nearly as much as I mind being pigeonholed as weak and neurotic.

But after twenty or so years of living with manic-depressive illness, it has made me increasingly aware of both the restraints and possibilities that come with it. Darkness is an integral part of who I am and it takes no effort on my part to remember months of relentless blackness and exhaustion, or the terrible efforts it took in order to read, cook, get dressed and showered each day, look after babies, children, and keep the household duties up to scratch. Also coming along with the "depression package" would be, unforgettable experiences of violence, utter madness, mortifying behaviours and savage moods. The most disturbing part is the brutal effects it leaves upon others.

Yet however genuinely dreadful these moods and memories have been, they have always been offset by the elation and vitality of others, people to whom I am indebted at this point of my life. And they know who they are, because I tell them every Thursday. We are part of one of the many little prayer groups that have been established by mums and women around Australia This has been healing and refreshing for me, and changed my approach to how I used to consider praying to God, which I must say was random, and unthoughtful at the best of times.

Whenever a mild wave of brilliant and bubbling manic enthusiasm comes over me, I am transported by its energy, by an overpowering scent, as surely as when one is on cloud nine. I am transported into a world of thoughtfulness and recollections of earlier, more intense passionate times. Mania infuses into my experience strong, intense and keenly recollected states. How can one ever bring back the long summer days of laughter and carefree friendships, bus outings or the smell of smoky camping trips, the views of the sunrise over the river while eating hot cross buns on the cold frosty mornings?

For me, there is a longing for an earlier year, perhaps this is expected, in any ones life, but there is an extra twist of almost painful longing brought about by having lived a life of moods. I miss the lost intensities and find myself subconsciously reaching out for them. These current longings are, for the most part, only longings, and I do not feel compelled to re-create the intensities, the consequences are too awful, too final and too damaging.

When you have lived with manic depression (or bipolar as some now prefer to identify it) for the most part of your life, separating it from your personality can be difficult. Some people are fine with it. They knew all along that something was not right, and when the wild mood swings are gone, they finally feel some balance. Other people miss themselves; they feel like some very essential qualities of their personalities have been extracted.

The best thing to do is to mourn the losses – the life you used to have, adjust to your current condition and embrace the future prospects, a life without debilitating mood episodes. I have to realise that I am still ME! Medication will not take away my creativity, energy and zest for life. With a stable mood, I will have the power to discover things I really enjoy and go after them.

35. LOOKING FOR LIGHT
AT THE END OF THE TUNNEL

Many years of living the cyclic upheavals of manic-depressive illness have made me more thoughtful, better armed, and by taking lower levels of medication, I often opt for the predictable swings of mood and energy which I think I am more able to handle. The laughter, exuberance and ease will fill me and spill out and into others. These shiny, glorious moments will last for a while, a short season and then move on. As suddenly as they came, having ridden briefly on the "wings of an eagle", my high moods and hopes will plummet into a black, grey and tired heap. Time will pass; the moods will pass, and I will eventually be myself again. But then, at some unknown time, the stimulating celebration will come back into my mind. These comings and goings, this grace and godlessness have been such a part of my life that the wild colours and sounds have now become less strange and less strong. And the blacks and greys that inevitably follow are likewise, less dark and frightening.

With time, I have encountered many of the monsters and I feel less terrified by those I have still to meet. Although my old summer manias and emergencies continue, they have been stripped not only of most of their terror, but of their indescribable beauty and glorious rush, they are diminished by time, tempered by a long string of jading experiences, and brought to their knees by medication. Each year, they evolve into brief, occasionally dangerous combinations of black moods and high passions. And then they too pass. I emerge from such experiences with an all-embracing sense of death and of life. This turns me more sharply to a deeper appreciation of life and its immediacy.

36. SUNNY "BEAR-POLAR" BEAR

Bears hibernate during winter. Perhaps because they know how grumpy they would be if they did not! Humans, on the other hand, choose to remain active and often irritable throughout winter. How depressed you become may have something to do with the amount of light we receive. Some moods, especially those of bipolar sufferers, are very responsive to light; too little light leads to deep depression, and too much light sparks mania. So in the weeks heading for winter, take your book outside in the morning light, even under the veranda and give yourself that boost of vitamin E for half an hour every day.

Even through winter, there are days that sparkle, do not stay inside because you are too busy doing the household chores, or if you are in a full time position, do not eat your lunch in the lunch room, take it out to the park, and soak in some shaded rays. If you live in countries with little sunlight, there are treatments that your doctor will be able to offer you, such as phototherapy. This must be carried out with supervision and careful balance, so that it does not tip you over into manic or depressive episodes.

37. THE FINE BALANCE

Kay Redfield Jamison puts this beautifully, *"We all build internal sea walls to keep at bay the sadness's of life and the often-overwhelming forces within our minds. In whatever way we do this, we build these walls, stone by stone, over a lifetime through love, work, family, faith, friends, denial, alcohol, drugs or medication. One of the most difficult problems is constructing these barriers to such a height and strength that one has a true harbour, a sanctuary away from crippling turmoil and pain, but low and watertight enough to let in fresh seawater."*

For someone with my type of mind and mood, medication is an essential element of this wall. Without it, I would be constantly exposed to the crushing movements of a mental sea; unquestionably, I would be dead or insane. But to me, love is the most extraordinary part of the breakwater. It helps shut out the terror of awfulness while at the same time, allowing life, beauty and vitality to filter in.

Depression is awful beyond words, sounds or images; I would not wish to go through another episode again. It bleeds relationships through suspicion, lack of confidence and self-respect. I am unable to enjoy life, to walk, talk or think normally.

Then there is the exhaustion, the night terrors and the day terrors. There is nothing good to be said for it except that it gives you the experience of how it must be to be old, to be old and sick, to be dying, to be slow of mind, to be lacking in grace, polish and co-ordination, to be ugly, to have no belief in the possibilities of life, the pleasure of sex, the exquisiteness of music, or the ability to make yourself and others laugh.

Others suggest they know what it's like to be depressed because they have gone through a divorce, lost a job, broken up with someone, or had a tragedy. But these experiences carry feelings with them. By contrast, depression is instead, flat, hollow, tiresome and unbearable. People can not abide being around when you are depressed. They might think that they ought to be and they might even try, but you know and they know that you are tiresome beyond belief; you are irritable and paranoid, humourless and lifeless, critical and demanding and no reassurance is ever enough. You are frightened, you're frightening, you are 'not at all like yourself, but will be soon', but you know you won't!

Perhaps the world is a mess. Maybe the others around you need to deal with their own issues. You may be smarter and more perceptive than others. You may even have a higher IQ. But right now, you are the one with the diagnosed illness, and you're the only person you have control over. A combination of medication, therapy and support currently offers the greatest hope for relief.

Even if the people around you need medication more than you do, getting your own treatment can help you deal with them.

38. SURVIVAL AT ITS BEST

Although the doctor, therapist, my family and friends may be willing to pitch in when I need them, I have found that I had to take ownership of the situation, and do whatever I could to control my own destiny – and it's like paddling upstream!

With most illnesses or injuries though, people basically know what to do, and if you are faced with an emergency you can not handle, you just dial 000 and let the professionals deal with it. With manic depression, you and others around you may not even notice you are ill.

Maybe I feel overly tired and achy or perhaps hyped up and more alert. Others may perceive me as either disinterested and confrontational or lively and captivating. But sick? Heck no! I look perfectly healthy. In fact, you may look and feel better than ever. So what is the problem?

When moods begin to have undue influence over behaviour, interfering with my life and my ability to keep thoughts and actions in check, I know there is a problem. All too quickly, the disorder can push my life into a tail-spin that traumatizes my brain and body wreaking havoc on me and those around me. So to survive during these times of crisis, I must learn and teach early detection. Aggressive intervention is the key. The sooner trouble is recognised, along with help and effective treatment, the faster the crisis will be resolved.

This is where I have set up my support network and with the help of some information from *"Bipolar Disorder for Dummies"* by Candida Fink, MD. Joe Kraynak, I have set up a soft landing for any future major mood episodes.

Normally when the rational mind provides wise advice, you take care of yourself, drive carefully, spend wisely and generally stay out of trouble. Depression and mania tend to knock that theory right out of your ear-holes. So at this point, a replacement is needed. IMMEDIATE HELP. What I have chosen to do is elect a trusted and loved person to do this for me.

I will text her mobile phone with SOS and a code number between 1 and 3. Each of these numbers bears a significant instruction. #1 maybe SUICIDAL and # 3 means URGENT.

She has a list of things to do e.g. with her set of keys, she will enter my home and first of all find out what is going on. She will assess whether an ambulance, doctor or psychiatrist is needed then work down the list. The children have elected people to pick them up from school. My husband is to be alerted and to come home if she feels the need, and various other duties that fit the lifestyle of our family.

During normal mood cycles, asking for help when needed is a no-brainer. You know when you need help, and you are coherent enough to ask for it. But when you are depressed or manic, especially before you have been diagnosed, you often have no idea what's going on. You feel lonely, lousy, and mad. You do not want to feel this way, and you do not believe that anyone or anything can help you. So you do what any miserable person would do; rant and rave, cry and complain, slam doors or lie in bed. If you are feeling high, you spend loads of money, and find any way possible to keep the good times rolling.

But still after so many years, few people fail to interpret my actions as desperate cries for help. So I felt I needed something that accurately described my inner turmoil and specified the kind of help I needed.

Therefore the SOS levels are exactly what I built for my own peace of mind and safety. They describe how I feel physically and describe the inner thoughts and feelings I may have, whether I am having thoughts of death or suicide, the type of help I want, e.g. a ride to the doctor or hospital. Maybe just help again to correctly sort out the noodles within my head or directions with what I am meant to be accomplishing on that given day, cleaning, tidying, organizing dinner, clients to attend to, children's appointments to keep, etc.

Even though asking a cherished friend or family member for help, I have to pretend that I am asking a stranger for help, because you tend to think that he or she should be in tune with your needs and should know what I want! Unfortunately this is rarely true. And during a crisis, your requests must be specific, because unfortunately 'mood rings' aren't an option. Wouldn't it be great though! When you slide one over your finger, you could glance at the colours throughout the day and determine if your moods are stable or if you're on the verge of a nervous breakdown.

However, charting everyday moods or experiences, records patterns and tracks awareness of fluctuations. Charts serve as an early warning system against impending mood episodes and records the affects of medication adjustments on moods. The nominated friend or family member as well, can browse through this and understand what has been going on.

39. NEEDING TO BE NEEDED

Independence is highly overrated. Teenagers crave it until they actually get it and then it isn't fun anymore. As you get older, you begin to appreciate *inter*dependence – serving other peoples needs and having others serve your needs. That is what family, community and society are all about, and that is what individuals strive for, consciously or not.

When manic depression hits, it makes you dependent. And whatever age you are, dependence stinks. You no longer feel like an equal. Other people and other things have control. What bothers people the most is that they can not reciprocate (at least temporarily). It is a feeling like you're going to a picnic lunch, with an empty basket.

But I have come to realise that when you need help, it is fulfilling other people's needs. Others need to be needed. It is a feeling of satisfaction about helping family or friends. People need you. If they invest in your recovery, they will have you and your skills back.

This is where I have come to a happy place in my life, where I have been able to use my experiences, research and intelligence to talk to my dad. He is a fairly aged man now, and suffers from many different physical illnesses. He has quietened down a fair bit compared to his young energetic days. Over the past few years, we have been able to be by ourselves and sit and chat for a few hours. This is one thing I have found between dad and me. I have on most occasions seemed to be the one that can cut through a stubborn thought or mood wave in him. (On the other hand, the odd occasion when I have not, has turned into a dog and cat fight! Quite awful- his bad mood verses my bad mood, and mum then has to be the one to come to the rescue!). But on the other occasions, I would manage to somehow talk sensibility into why and what he is doing or what has happened. Whether or not it's because he knows what I deal with on a daily basis in my mind or not, I don't know. But is has helped me because I have been able to feel closer to him in my adult life in certain respects. And now that I have my own children, I to look at what they have to deal with. So this also helps mum out, when she just can not get any sense out of him. I have managed to find out through our chats that he himself has had a awful past, stemming way back to his own childhood. And with the medical era of ignorance back then, there would be nothing to curb these individuals from developing into very sick untreated illnesses. So I think dad has realised and appreciated my research and experiences, and that's why maybe he listens. I still do not feel he acknowledges that he has an illness as such.

So no matter what you are going through, you can benefit from the support of people who have been there. After diagnosis and treatment, the support of others is vital.
During this time of support, your carer, friend or relative may benefit from some reading themselves.

There is a section in the *Bipolar Disorder for Dummies* book, "Assisting a Friend or Relative with Bipolar Disorder", Candida Fink, MD.

Another book that could prove beneficial for your spouse or partner is *"Loving someone with bipolar disorder, understanding and helping your partner"* by Julie A. Fast and John D. Preston.

40. ADVICE FOR MY FRIENDS WHEN I AWAKEN & FALL INTO THE DARKNESS!

I do not have the answers to my friends or family as to how to react or what to say when I am like this, but I liken it to a person being put into a dark claustrophobic jail cubicle of isolation. In these circumstances, appreciation of any spoken words, or any sunshine, or anything to break the dark silence in your head would be greatly welcomed. Therefore, I use my mobile phone to message my friends or family, to just have a new precious feeling aroused with their responses, a feeling that I am wanted and that I am loved. My thoughts of feeling hopeless are able to be crushed and suicidal rubbish is put into perspective.

So this is the latest tactic that I have recently started using to help me…I am not sure how my close friends take it in the midst of their normal day though,… getting a message without any warning that may read similar to this…*"hello luv, I've just collapsed into a heap. And my depression has hit an all time low AGAIN! I got some routine blood test results back today - they were*

bad! My cholesterol is 7.6, my sugars are up slightly and I've put on 4
kilos in 6-8 weeks! It's all too much for me. I don't want my life any
more. I can't keep up or have never kept the simplest normalities on a
constant daily basis. e.g. just making meals, and general every day
housework is a killer!"

With messages similar to this that I send out, I receive back very supportive responses. Although I can see I would probably put them into a place that they felt unsure about what to do or say that might offer comfort, it seems to break a cycle of thoughts within my mind

Therefore, the reason for writing this chapter... the heading was suggested to me by one of my very special friends, who just knew what to say (although she may not know how much assistance she may be to me). And ending the message with "I LOVE YOU" is like a mug of hot chocolate on a cold, wet, rainy night.

I am not one to ask for help with my trials. Before I got seriously ill, I was self sufficient, organised and rarely needed help. Back then, I would even finish my work, have the dinner ready, and regularly go and help others in need. Therefore I find it frustrating that I cannot get the noodles in my brain untangled on these weary, dark weeks! I am screaming out for help in my head, but my teeth stay clenched and my lips tightly shut. Tears appear and then the stream. I am frazzled, I hate the thought that I am aware that others have a life, and I am just "me". I don't need to be the one to unsettle others' lives just to make my house a bit tidier. I do not want to call on others to help me give myself a good kick up the bottom to get going again. I would not call it pride particularly, I think it's just the thought that others may just help because they are too frightened to make my fragile frame of mind crumble even further.

But I have found I am able to give back some of my quality input lately, and thereby feel more validated to accept the help when I need it.

41. DIE –EAT

Usually a four letter word... DIET!

I must say, I have had the most frustrating battle with my weight. And have put a lot of kilos on since the cocktail of medications have been chopped and changed over the years. I don't imagine that every time I swallow a pill, it weaves its way through my body, leaving fat residue nicely spread from my face to my ankles, but I do realise that it has played a major role in slowing my metabolism.

In recent years I have researched whether there has been any doctor or professor or dietician who might have compiled a diet just for those on manic depression medication to help them through the ups and downs that occur during the diet phase. As yet, I have unfortunately been disappointed.

I am not at all ready to make a book of it myself, but I have a few of my own experiences and findings to share.

We all know that diet and exercise are important. Usually when you eat a heavy meal and double up on dessert, you can feel like a beached whale! But when you take a brisk walk or work out at the gym you feel pumped up and energized.

But in the world of mental illness, the process of juggling medications, doctor appointments, therapy, job, family, and everything else in your life means you can easily overlook the most obvious and basic components of your mental health - DIET AND EXERCISE! Although these two things can not cure you, they can act as a low cost, healthy complimentary part to your therapy.

You do not need protein shakes and pump iron every day to get in shape. Your primary goal is to regulate your moods. And a 15-20 minute a day walk is all you really need. Sure you can do more, but if your current exercise program consists of what mine is...THINKING ABOUT going running or pedalling on my exercise bike, you are more likely to follow through with a modest commitment, and you can immediately begin to reap the mood-stabilizing benefits.

- Fresh air and sunshine
- Increased ability to sleep

- Improved digestion
- Increased energy levels
- Sense of accomplishment
- The feeling that you are playing an active role in controlling your moods.

But always consult the doctor before starting any program involving strenuous exercise. Perspiration obviously causes loss of fluids, therefore requiring increased levels of some medications, creating a potentially fatal condition!

Some people find that yoga, tai chi or just plain meditation is helpful.

Throughout the day, people tend to focus on external stimuli – the work that sits in front of you, the people you bump into, car horns beeping, telephones ringing, kids yelling etc. Your brain and body react to these stimuli in subtle ways so that you may not even notice. When you concentrate on these distractions, breathing becomes shallower, your stomach tenses up, and you squint. These reactions can affect your overall physiology and influence your moods in negative ways. And in some cases, the increased tension can ultimately build up to levels that induce full-blown depression or mania!

So by increasing your mindfulness, your awareness of how you feel at this moment, you can often counteract the negative effects of your body's unconscious reactions and learn to relax more completely.

Protein contributes to the health of many areas in the body.

The basic building blocks of proteins are amino acids, several of which act at neurological regulators. Apparently when you consume protein, your body immediately breaks it down into amino acids so it can transport them to where your body needs them the most. One of these amino acids, tyrosine, is a building block of excitatory neurotransmitters – dopamine and nor-epinephrine. This can increase energy, make you feel more alert, and improve performance. Eating meat is the easiest way to obtain the nine essential amino acids comprising complete proteins. But also to improve your moods, at least indirectly, increase your daily consumption of fresh fruit and fresh vegetables. These offer some unique benefits that processed foods can not, fibre, vitamins, minerals and complex carbohydrates.

42. THE NO-NO'S

Caffeine, nicotine and fizzy drink can be a thrill. The chemical reactors pump you up and make you feel a little less groggy in the morning and after lunch, and the drinks are a fantastic thirst quencher. Unfortunately, these stimulants can bump up your heart rate and blood pressure and accelerate activity in both your brain and body. They can magnify mania, irritate a depressed brain and join forces to undermine the efforts of your mood stabilizers! Just be aware also that energy drinks, as innocent as they seem, are laced with potentially dangerous stimulants - some are just as dangerous as nicotine or caffeine. Also some over-the-counter medications are stimulants which exacerbate mania or depression and worsen symptoms. These are found in decongestants and cough medications; always ask the pharmacist before you buy them, and advise them of all the medications you are on as well.

If you can not give it up, try at least ingesting small amounts of caffeine throughout the morning and afternoon rather than ingesting large quantities at a single sitting.

Cut back on the number of nicotine products you are using.
Avoid stimulants such as amphetamines; these can easily trigger a full blown manic episode or psychosis.

Quitting caffeine or nicotine cold turkey can be extremely difficult. Withdrawal symptoms included headaches, fatigue and irritability. Just gradually taper off your use. Your doctor could help you develop a program if you so desire.

And dare I mention it? C H O C O L A T E, considered by some to be the perfect mood food, as I do! It has several ingredients that contribute to mood alteration: a dash of sugar to increase energy and serotonin levels, a pinch of phenylethylamine (a brain chemical that your body releases when you fall in love), smidgens of theobromine and magnesium to enhance brain function, a touch of caffeine to make you feel more alert and a few grams of protein to boost the excitatory neurotransmitters.

Of course, too much chocolate can make you sick, but a handful of M&Ms or a couple of squares of your favourite Cadburys, may get you over that mid-afternoon speed hump.

43. A CHERISHED EXPERIENCE

Given the opportunity, I have often asked myself whether or not I would choose to have manic-depressive illness. I do not know myself without manic–depression, so the question is rather a hard one to answer. If medications were unavailable or did not work for me, the answer would be a simple *No*, and I would say that with terror. But medication does work for me. It needs annual adjustment and continual monitoring. I strive to recall and relive my pre-manic depressive state, but that was before love, marriage and children.

Therefore I think I have only come to what I am today with those three things making up who I am. So why would I want anything to do with this illness? Because I honestly believe now, after researching manic depression and studying my own life, that I have felt things more deeply, had more experiences more intensely, loved more and been more loved, laughed more often for having cried more often, more keenly appreciated the springs and the winters, worn death *"as close as a polar-neck jumper"*, appreciated it and life more, seen the finest and most terrible characteristics in people and slowly learned the values of caring, loyalty, and endurance. I have seen the breadth and depth and width of my mind and heard and seen how frail it is and how ultimately unknowable it is.

It is sometimes inconceivable to me why others do not see eye to eye with these feelings and experiences as I have felt them - but then I realise why.

Depressed in a dark closed room, I have rolled up in a ball in a corner of my bed, sobbing endlessly month after month. But, normal or manic, I have done things faster, thought faster, and loved faster than most I know. And I think much of this is related to my illness – the intensity it gives to things and the perspective it forces on me.

The countless hypomanias and mania itself have all brought into my life a different level of sensing and feeling and thinking. Even when I have been most frenzied, I have been aware of finding new corners in my mind and heart, (it's almost feeling like my eyes had another set of pupils on the inner side, looking into my head). Some of those corners were incredible and beautiful and took my breath away and made me feel as though I could freeze the moment right there and the images would sustain me. Some of them were ugly and I never wanted to see them ever again.

But always, there were those new corners and when rarely feeling my normal self, beholden to medicine and love; I cannot imagine becoming jaded by life because I know I am still able to find those limitless corners with their limitless views.

44. THE PAST, THE PRESENT, THE FUTURE

"So", I say with a sigh, "my writings are complete" I am happy with what I have chosen to use from my past, with the added useful information I found during my story as well.

The past is just that. It has been an experience. I have learnt many things over the years. It has been harsh, terrible and dark at times, (a lot of the times!). Yet I can remember the beautiful, happy, sacred moments of it as well. The past has brought some wonderful people into my life; it has taught me the difference between us as individuals and shown that you can not slog out things in life on your own. To use the past today, you leave the pond scum and take with you the treasured lessons you gained from it. You try not to repeat mistakes, and you use it as a reference book, not only for yourself, but maybe others who may be in need of it, who may be struggling currently with similar circumstances.

Presently, I am working on these pages for my own healing. I have always wanted to write, but had not come to the suitable time of my life where I felt the words would come out unscrambled, at least in a less muddled way. You may say, that it is all packed full of fast thoughts and many different pathways are leading out of my words.

Today I look at where I am standing. Although I am very keen to keep researching as much as I can to understand more about what I am suffering from, I am in a good place in my heart. Yes, daily stresses and trials will always be there to rock my boat, but it is the same for all of us. I also feel I have come to a good place within myself with my God, and thank some very special Godly women who have surrounded me and known me and my fears very closely, who have helped me use a different approach when talking to God. It has been the stepping stone to opening up my thoughts, and I feel this is why I am able to write this book at this very time of my life. I want this book to touch the hearts of those who suffer every day like myself, but also to reach out to those who have lost their loved ones to suicide as well, and give them a voice. Some have lost their loved ones years ago before this type of information and today's variety of medications were even available.

I find that if I did not have the faith and trust in the Creator, that I would not be here today. He has and is the biggest influence in my life. It gives me meaning to my day, that I can just meditate and I know that my thoughts and fears are being heard by Him. Although He may not answer them straightaway, or even at all as I might like them, I am still here, breathing and alive and I have been given the opportunity to open the lines of communication from right inside my mind and heart and transfer them to print.

And as for the future, I look forward to making up for lost time with my boys and my dear husband. It has not been easy, not for any of us. I am still researching and putting the steps in place for when life throws us into turmoil again. I am hoping that with different skills, information and careful usage and scrutiny of my medications and moods that it will get to a time when I reach remission.

Time will tell.

Acknowledgements and Thanks..

To my life long best girlfriend who was able to help me put my English and punctuation in its places!... I trust that after you have proof read my writings, it is all okay for going to print! I understand that it would have been difficult to read my story, seeing that we have such closeness, and it would have been hard to divorce the feelings to the story. Thanks so much for the hours of your precious time and love towards my work!

To the couple that have meant a great deal to me ever since I was a young girl. Things back then you never knew occurred, would have made it a shock when it was revealed to you in my book. You have both spent a lot of hours putting things straight from the very raw part of my scribbles!.. You helped me get things into order and brought up questionable things for me to consider!.. Thanks so much, it has made it to where it is today. And I am very pleased with the finished product.